The Astrology of Great Gay Sex

The Astrology of Great Gay Sex

The Ultimate Guide to Finding Mr. Right and Avoiding Mr. Wrong

Myrna Lamb

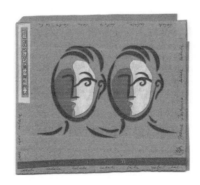

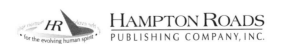

HAMPTON ROADS
PUBLISHING COMPANY, INC.

Cover design by Jane Hagaman
Cover art: Twins © Roy McMahon/zefa/Corbis; astrological chart © 2008 Visual Language®
Interior photography © ImageZoo Media Inc.

Hampton Roads Publishing Company, Inc.
1125 Stoney Ridge Road
Charlottesville, VA 22902

434-296-2772
fax: 434-296-5096
e-mail: hrpc@hrpub.com
www.hrpub.com

If you are unable to order this book from your local
bookseller, you may order directly from the publisher.
Call 1-800-766-8009, toll-free.

Library of Congress Cataloging-in-Publication Data
Lamb, Myrna, 1942-
  The astrology of great gay sex : the ultimate guide to finding Mr. Right
and avoiding Mr. Wrong / Myrna Lamb.
     p. cm.
  Summary: "Gay men answer a series of questions about their sexual
preferences. The results are compiled by zodiac sign and show significant
correspondences within a given sign. Designed to help gay men find the
perfect partner"--Provided by publisher.
  ISBN-13: 978-1-57174-575-0 (alk. paper)
  1. Astrology and sex. 2. Gay men--Miscellanea. I. Title.
  BF1729.H66L36 2008
  133.5'83067662--dc22

                              2007052775

ISBN 978-1-57174-575-0
10 9 8 7 6 5 4 3 2 1
Printed on acid-free paper in Canada

This book is dedicated to three men.

Tom Seers

In Memoriam
Gifted astrologer, friend, and mentor, without
whom this book would never have been started.

Ron Nelson

Quintessential Virgo, a man who embodies the meaning
of friendship—steadfast, patient, ever-present—without
whom this book would never have been finished.

Robert Lamb

Extraordinary artist, husband, and soul mate without whose love
and encouragement this book would be missing its heart.

CONTENTS

Aries
The Ram
March 21–April 19

PAGE **1**

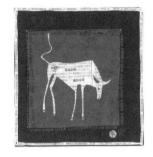

Taurus
The Bull
April 20–May 20

PAGE **17**

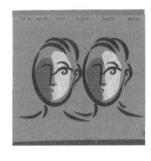

Gemini
The Twins
May 21–June 20

PAGE **33**

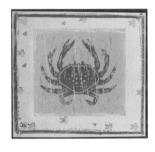

Cancer
The Crab
June 21–July 22

PAGE **49**

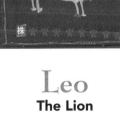

Leo
The Lion
July 23–August 22

PAGE **65**

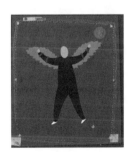

Virgo
The Virgin
August 23–September 22

PAGE **81**

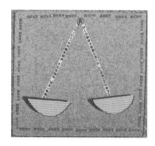

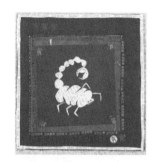

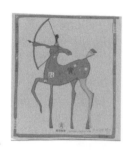

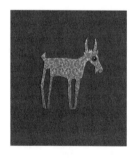

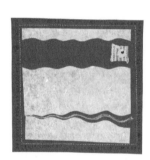

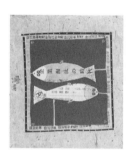

Acknowledgments

I wish to extend my appreciation to:

My literary agent Bill Gladstone of Waterside Productions and to Ming Russell, with appreciation for their commitment to this project and for their excellent representation.

Jeff Gellman of MIKO Exoticwear for getting me started in the distribution of the Sex Survey and to Options of Rhode Island for promoting that questionnaire.

And to Jakob for occupying himself and letting me work.

A special debt of gratitude is due to the hundreds of men who gave of their time to complete the sex questionnaires that form the basis for this book.

Introduction

What's inside This Book?

Sex and lots of it.

More than 1,400 people completed a sex survey leading to this book.

Quotes from hundreds of men have been included. Their explicit comments and generous contributions made it possible to write this very different kind of astrology book. Firsthand, learn what your lover likes, dislikes, wants, and fantasizes about in the world of sex.

How to Use This Book

For chapters 1 through 12, go to the table of contents to find your birthday* and your Sun Sign, your lover's sign, or the sign for anyone else you might want to check out. When you turn to that chapter, feel free to open to any page and read whatever parts interest you. The way the book is laid out, in question and answer format, there is no need to read the chapter from beginning to end. Most pages have short vignettes in boxes. These are the sexual fantasies and memories from hundreds of men who completed the questionnaire.

The questions come from the sex questionnaire and all the answers have been taken directly from the completed surveys. Frequently, you will find repetition among the answers. Repetition shows the consistency with which people of a given Sun Sign responded to a question.

Sexual Compatibility through the Zodiac

The second part of this book describes the way each Sign relates to every other. It begins with Aries partnered with Aries, then with Taurus, with Gemini, and continues all the way through Pisces with Pisces.

---

*If you were born on the first day or the last day of a Sign, you may not be sure which chapter to read. There are many websites online that will let you know which of the two is your actual Sun Sign, or you may write to me and I'll check it for you. Go to www.MyrnaLamb.com.

On a few occasions, there are sections that seem a little contradictory. That is because some Signs bring out certain traits in an individual, but put that same man with another Sun Sign and the result can be quite different.

Premise of This Book

The Astrology of Great Gay Sex began with a simple premise. The Sun Sign is the most basic and deepest level of the astrology of personality. Sex is among the most basic of human urges. It follows that the characteristics of one's Sun Sign should relate to that individual's sexual behaviors and preferences.

To test that relationship, I devised a sex questionnaire and asked people to fill it out anonymously. The consistency of the answers received from people of the same Sign was remarkable. For instance, in answer to the question, "How do you feel about public displays of affection?" all Scorpios, who are known for being secretive, reported that they do not enjoy them. *"I am not interested. I do not want to see it and I'm not into showing."*

Another example, Gemini, the Sign of Communication, when asked, "What do you like to do on a date?" always included liking to talk. *"Most of all I want to have fun and especially share good conversation."* "[I like] *sitting in a café and talking."*

The Questionnaire

The questionnaire consists of seven sections covering an individual's attitudes toward sex and relationships, sexual behaviors, fantasies, memories of significant encounters, and interest in sexual fetishes. A copy of the survey is included at the back of the book. Filling it out and comparing answers with your lover could do wonders to enrich and broaden your sex life.

The questionnaire was distributed through my website, advertisements, and announcements in newspapers and on radio programs. I also handed it out at fetish fairs and Pride Parades and gave it to my astrology clients.

Who This Book Is For

This book is for men of all ages, whether in new or longstanding relationships, who want to know more about how to make their sex lives more fulfilling. What better way to learn than to read your lover's own words?

Using What You've Learned

Some men, even those in committed relationships, are reticent about telling their lovers how to please them. In the pages of this book, you'll find out. For instance, when a Capricorn man is asked, "How do you demonstrate affection for your partner?" He reports that he shows his caring by helping his partner, quietly participating, without waiting to be asked and without drawing attention to himself.

"I try to maintain the house the way he likes it, and I give him space."

"I do things for him that he does not like to do, such as his laundry."

"I am attentive. I get things for him and help out, however he needs."

Clearly he would appreciate a partner who treats him this thoughtfully in return.

In some cases, one partner wants to explore that sexual territory existing beyond the bounds of mainstream sex, also called "vanilla" sex. *The Astrology of Great Gay Sex* will help you determine what direction your lover might accept and what areas are apt to be taboo.

Learning about your lover's fantasies can add considerably to your sex life. Fantasies are safe, an opportunity to think anything without breaking laws or taboos. For example, Aquarius envisions aggressive scenes with multiple partners and activities ranging from double penetration to rape. *"Gang rape with cowboys. . . . I want sex with a police officer. . . . I imagine sex while getting a tattoo, being pierced, while having a massage, or at work."* Many people are not interested in acting out their fantasies, but introducing some element of it, a costume or sex toy, even talking about images from it, during a sexual encounter will spice things up for your lover.

The Elements: Fire, Earth, Air, and Water

The Signs of the zodiac fall into four categories. They are FIRE, EARTH, AIR, and WATER. Within each element, there are three Signs, and they have some qualities in common. If your lover is a Taurus, it may also be of interest to scan the Virgo and Capricorn chapters. Also, when it comes to compatibility, generally Fire Signs and Air Signs are harmonious, and Water and Earth Signs suit each other well.

FIRE (ARIES, LEO, SAGITTARIUS)

The Fire Signs are perhaps the most active sexually. Their passion is intense, but sex may be quick. For Aries, sex can be about showing off how good he is, especially at kissing and oral sex. Leo is never to be outdone at anything and certainly that includes sexual functioning. Sagittarius—well even the symbol of Sagittarius, half man/half horse, speaks to his desire to prove his animal magnetism. With all three, praise is a vital stimulus.

EARTH (TAURUS, VIRGO, CAPRICORN)

The Earth Signs are the earthiest signs in respect to the range of their sexuality. They love to touch, taste, and smell. Taurus likes sex that lasts longer and may want to touch all parts of his lover's body. Virgo may be more systematic in his approach, though also open to experimentation. Capricorn is perhaps even more open to extreme sex. But all three of these Earth Signs are very physical. Food turns them on and material goods are important to them.

AIR (GEMINI, LIBRA, AQUARIUS)

The Air Signs are more cerebral than the other Sun Signs, and they seek intimacy through sex. It's the man who has plenty to say who scores with him. Gemini is at once participant and observer, stimulated by his partner's responses as much as by the sensations he himself is feeling. For Libra, anticipation is a major part in setting the stage for sex, and for Aquarius, trying a range of behaviors is important in his quest to feel things intensely.

WATER (CANCER, SCORPIO, PISCES)

The Water Signs are likely to be the most passionate in terms of the expression of emotion in sex. Cancer's sexuality grows out of a need to nurture, Scorpio's out of the need to be desired, and Pisces's comes from idealized romantic passion. All three Signs are extremely sexual and sensitive to their partner's feelings. Setting the stage for sex and picking locales near water are surefire triggers to put Water Signs in the mood. Getting turned on results from a sense of emotional closeness.

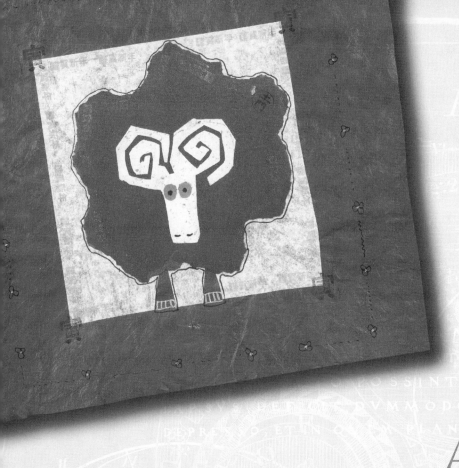

Aries
THE RAM

March 21 through April 19

FIRE SIGN ARIES is impulsive, assertive, and in some ways a perpetual child. Ruler of the head and the features of the face, the Ram loves oral sex. To satisfy Aries in lovemaking, that which is indispensable above all else is passionate kissing.

What he says: "Often, when I see someone, I turn it into something sexual. I wonder if he has a big dick. It makes my heart jump. I want to rip his clothes off."

"If you wanna know if he loves you so, it's in his kiss. . . . Oh yeah it's in his kiss (that's where it is)."
—"The Shoop Shoop Song," lyrics by Rudy Clark

The Aries Man
in His Own Words

"While sipping Chardonnay in front of my fireplace, my friend and I began to kiss and play. He didn't want to remove his underwear because he hadn't been with a man before. I had him lie back to relax, took a mouth full of wine, and slowly let the warm liquid drip from my mouth through his underwear over his dick. He thought the sensation was incredible, then removed his wet briefs. We had a wonderful sexual encounter."

Attraction and Dating an Aries

WHAT ATTRACTS YOU TO SOMEONE?

Since this Sign rules the head and facial features, Aries always notices a man's lips and smile. In fact, he is quite specific about what turns him on, and hair plays an important part.

"I love hairy men, hairy chest, legs. At the beach, if I see a hairy guy, what a turn on! Another guy with a perfect physique can walk by . . . and nothing. Give me the chubby guy that's hairy."

"The man who turns me on has high energy, is hairy, strong and clean looking, of average height, weighs 185 to 210 pounds, and has a one- to two-inch-thick cock."

"The size of a guy's dick doesn't mean a lot to me. But when I have sex with a new partner that's the first thing I check out. What does it look like; what does it feel like? I've seen some weird ones."

WHAT MIGHT TURN YOU OFF?

He is, in some respects, a perpetual child, and play is important to him. Therefore, a man who lacks a sense of humor or is overly serious will turn him off. In addition, as he loves to kiss, poor dental hygiene is an absolute negative.

"Too serious a personality, being too thin or too tall. I like people shorter than I am. Maybe that puts me in a more dominant position."

"Bad teeth are a big turnoff; someone who isn't intelligent; a person who has no class."

"Piercings turn me right off. I call it shrapnel."

WHAT DO YOU ENJOY DOING ON A DATE?

Aries likes a lot of attention and appears to be quite sure of himself, but one of his boyish qualities is a touch of shyness. As a result, when he is first getting to know a man, he prefers dating activities that divert attention, such as going to a movie or an amusement park.

"I like doing something physical: walk, go to the beach, and silly things; leaving silly token gifts for him."

"I prefer to do something new, cheap, and exciting; bowling, miniature golf; music, see a show, or just take a walk. I'm turned off by the generic dinner and movie scenarios."

"I enjoy going to hockey games, football games, movies, a play, the beach; having dinner and taking a walk."

"Sharing a meal, whether home cooked or at a restaurant. Food is an easy, comfortable way to engage in conversation. I think food is very sexual."

ARE YOU FLIRTATIOUS?

Fun-loving Aries has a flirtatious quality, whether talking with men, women, or children. He sees flirtation as harmless fun.

MEMORIES

"Drove a guy home. He started kissing me then undressed me in the car. It was very aggressive. We went to fuck. I was so excited I didn't last at all and he wet my ass and balls cumming quickly. That drove me to a fast climax. Dominant men in leather boots usually make me cum too fast."

"One of the best was when my partner came up behind me in a very aggressive way and I obliged him. He took what he needed."

"I am very flirtatious. Flirt, walk away, come back, and flirt again. I'll flirt with all people. I'm just being playful."

"I am the biggest flirt on the face of the earth because I like people. It means nothing more than that, really."

ARE YOU JEALOUS?

In much the way that a child wants Daddy's full attention, so Aries expects to be the focal point for his lover. So even though he admits to being a flirt himself, he does not tolerate such behavior from his partner.

"Of course I'm jealous—I'm gay."

"Unfortunately, I'm very predatory; yes I am jealous."

"By nature I'm jealous, but I strive to abolish it immediately. Jealousy isn't part of who I want to be."

A FANTASY

"I have several . . . dick in my mouth and ass, eating clean-shaven ass holes, hands rubbing firm bodies, bodies all over me, eating sweet cum . . . being fed a long dick down my throat . . . sucking off a swim or basketball team. Fist fucking a smooth body, many beautiful men standing over me, cumming all over me, shooting cum on my face and into my mouth."

HOW DO YOU FEEL ABOUT PUBLIC DISPLAYS OF AFFECTION?

He might dance in public, talk a little loudly, and express joy. But when it comes to showing his feelings for his partner, a little is wonderful, more than that is not.

"Public displays are fine within reason. I like people knowing that I am with someone special to me. That doesn't mean necking on a park bench, but holding hands, a hug. . . ."

"I love to see young gay men in love."

"I see nothing wrong with it, unless you're sticking your hands down each other's pants and being gross."

"Little acts are great, but make-out sessions that look like foreplay are too much."

Sexual Attitudes and Behaviors

● ●

HOW OFTEN DO YOU THINK ABOUT SEX, AND HOW OFTEN PER WEEK DO YOU WANT TO HAVE SEX?

Sex is never far from the surface of his mind, and he enjoys having sex four times weekly.

"Often when I see someone, I turn it into something sexual. I wonder if he has a big dick. It makes my heart jump. I want to rip his clothes off."

A MEMORY

"I connected with a guy via the Internet, and we met in a hotel room. He was ten years older, muscular, a bit hairy and handsome, and had a beard. It wasn't long before he was fucking me so hard and nice that I came three times, without even touching my penis, just from receiving anal sex. My body was twitching and I was hyper-ventilating because it was so intense and enjoyable."

HOW LONG DO YOU LIKE TO SPEND HAVING SEX, AND HOW MUCH OF THAT TIME IS FOREPLAY? DO YOU ENJOY QUICKIES?

Aries likes sex sessions that last roughly twenty to thirty minutes. On occasion, he enjoys a marathon session, and he won't say "no" to a quickie.

"I don't care for long sex; some foreplay, kissing, then get right into the act; maybe ten to fifteen minutes foreplay, about twenty minutes start to finish."

"For me, sex is usually thirty minutes, with fifteen minutes of foreplay, and, yes, quickies are fine."

"Sometimes I like sex to last two to three hours with as much foreplay as possible, and quickies are fun as well."

WHAT TIME OF DAY DO YOU PREFER TO HAVE SEX?

Aries has a slight preference for sex at night but he isn't likely to turn sex down at any time of day. After all, he likes quickies. Why not enjoy that before, after, or in the middle of some other activity?

"I like sex right before bed or just after I get up, and I like being awakened for sex."

"Mornings are great but so are rainy afternoons."

HOW OFTEN PER WEEK DO YOU WANT TO HAVE SEX?

He enjoys sex seven times a week. If his partner has a lesser sex drive he'll content himself with sex two to four times weekly.

HOW OFTEN PER WEEK DO YOU MASTURBATE?

Most weeks he masturbates four times.

HOW LONG DO YOU WANT TO KNOW SOMEONE BEFORE GETTING SEXUAL?

Aries is known for being impulsive, and his reputation is on target in this area. It is an unusual Aries who wants to take his time. More often than not it's by becoming sexual that he knows whether he wants to pursue a relationship at all.

"Do I have to know them? Can't we just get sexual?"

"In the past I would have sex with someone immediately. Not anymore. I'm not in a hurry. I might wait 24 hours. It's hard for me to wait."

"I want to really know someone before getting intimate . . . perhaps a week or two."

MEMORIES

"A straight man delivered some furniture for me. We sat and talked a while. Then he began to get curious about sex with me. We started to touch each other. I undressed him and went down on him. He loved it. I loved it."

"He was thin, young, and attractive and kind enough to be considerate of my needs. He wanted to make me happy. The sex was nice, the comfort was nicer."

WHAT'S YOUR ATTITUDE TOWARD CASUAL SEX?

He is a risk taker and very lucky and trusts that luck when meeting someone new. Overall, he enjoys casual sex though he may not find it totally fulfilling.

"Casual sex isn't immoral, it's just not complete. I feel like I've engaged in it because of a lack of intimacy in my life, but it's stimulating, it's exciting."

"As long as you're safe, I see no harm in it. It's just sex."

"Casual sex is fine and I enjoy it very much, but in my heart I prefer a relationship."

DO YOU BELIEVE IN MONOGAMY?

He wants to be in a monogamous relationship, but to him that doesn't necessarily mean that he will have no outside sexual encounters.

"You can have many sexual partners and still have one love or soul mate."

"Yes, emotional monogamy, not sexual."

"Monogamy to me is commitment to provide emotional and financial support, to have security in the relationship. If a partner has sex outside the relationship, I don't want to know."

FANTASIES

"A repair man at the house asks to use the bathroom. He leaves the door open. After peeing he continues to stand there, stroking his cock to erection and asks me to join him."

"Being arrested by a cop and pleading to get out of it. He has to be sucked off and demands to have clean, spit-shined boots. After that he throws me over the hood of the car and fucks me."

DOES SEX HAVE A SPIRITUAL SIGNIFICANCE FOR YOU?

The core of the Aries disposition is loving and trusting. In a committed relationship, the sense of connection he feels to his lover has a unique quality. If he doesn't call it spiritual, he admits that it is special.

"If I feel connected to someone, sex has a spiritual significance as an extension of my loving him."

"It is a coming together of two spirits to enjoy something unique that we have to offer each other."

"I don't see sex as particularly spiritual, and yet loving and making love to that person is special."

ARE YOU COMFORTABLE INITIATING SEXUAL ACTIVITIES?

He is courageous and certainly willing to initiate. Still, the kid in him loves it when the other man shows enough regard and attention to approach him.

"In many relationships I was always the one to initiate sex and that didn't bother me. With my current partner we both do. I like spontaneous sex. I don't like setting a date to have sex. Anytime my partner wants sex, even if I wasn't in the mood, I'd get into it. I don't understand how anyone wouldn't."

HOW DO YOU COMMUNICATE TO YOUR PARTNER YOUR SEXUAL WANTS AND NEEDS?

Aries doesn't want to hurt his lover's feelings and uses gestures more than words to indicate what feels good sexually. He has a very direct nature and doesn't pick up subtleties easily, therefore, in bed Aries appreciates being told how to please.

"I don't communicate about sex very well. Sometimes I'm afraid I'll elicit the wrong stuff and if I do, I'll feel bad. Maybe I'll have asked for something I shouldn't have, but I'll move a hand . . . I'll acknowledge when something feels good. But there are times when someone's doing something to me, and he's obviously enjoying it, and I'll tolerate it even if I don't like it."

"When we are not having sex I talk about what I like. During sex, I grunt a lot. It is hard to talk when you are sucking and licking."

A MEMORY

"We met at the front door, kissing, groping and feeling up each other. As the kissing intensified we pulled off our clothes and rubbed our bodies together. The lights were dim and it was raining gently outside. Kicking off shoes and finally naked, I lay across the bed and invited him to come on board. There was lots of tongue, lots of tonguing on the body and moans of pleasure, oral then anal, and many different positions of fucking done with me by turns riding him and then being submissive."

DO YOU THINK OF YOURSELF AS BEING IN THE MAINSTREAM SEXUALLY, MORE EXPERIMENTAL, OR OPEN TO ANYTHING?

He is quite experimental, open to sexual activities including anal sex, dominance, and submission, using hot wax and ice cubes, exhibitionism, voyeurism, having sex in public places, and participating in orgies. He might use sex toys such as dildoes, vibrators, butt plugs. Very rarely he uses body clips and bondage accouterments.

In his fantasies Aries is usually submissive and his reservations about anonymous sex vanish.

HOW DO YOU DEMONSTRATE AFFECTION FOR YOUR PARTNER?

Aries, an active Fire Sign shows his regards with action. He does things for his lover to make him more comfortable, to make him laugh, to help him relax.

"I rub his shoulders, I cook him great dinners. Sometimes I clean up after him, give him flowers and small gifts. I help him any way I can."

"I like doing fun things, leaving silly notes for him and I like telling him that I am fond of him."

"I do whatever he wants me to do to make him happy."

The Five Senses

HOW IMPORTANT TO YOU IS THE SEXUAL ENVIRONMENT?

Aries is not a particularly fastidious Sign, but most of the time sensual lighting and at least some degree of cleanliness do matter to him.

"I couldn't stand a place that is disorderly or unclean."

"I watch my weight. If I am up five or ten pounds, I don't like much light in the room. If I am happy with my physique, then bright lights are just fine."

Aries also has a rash, impulsive side, which occasionally takes over in the heat of the moment.

"I've had sex in some of the grungiest toilets you've ever seen. Smell! But it was a turn-on, maybe because I was taking a risk, doing something in a place I shouldn't have been. It was exciting. It was an adventure."

A FANTASY

"While lying face down on a massage table, getting a great massage. Suddenly my arms and legs are bound with rope. My legs are spread wide and the therapist uses a lot of lube on my butt, fingers my prostate, and then uses a dildo very slowly."

WHERE DO YOU LIKE TO HAVE SEX?

Aries is a risk taker. Most often he has sex in the bedroom, but having sex outside it, in a car, on a rooftop, or in a club adds excitement.

"Mostly my bed, but anywhere indoors or outdoors as long as it is not cold."

"I like to have sex anywhere, in a car or outside in the woods. The best sex I ever had was on the kitchen floor with olive oil."

"Bed, living room, car, outside, almost anywhere if we are alone."

WHAT PUTS YOU IN THE MOOD FOR SEX?

Romance turns him on, "low lights, soft music, massage on my back and legs," though admittedly it's easy to get him started.

"Just seeing someone attractive puts me in the mood."

"I am always in the mood for sex, but candlelight is nice."

"I like him to touch my nipples and neck. I love his tongue in my ears. I love doing that to him too. . . . Hot oils . . . I enjoy doing and receiving rimming. I like his tongue in my groin area."

"Aroma of their bodies, physical contacts, the environment, sexy photos, but not porn."

WHAT'S YOUR ATTITUDE TOWARD PORNOGRAPHY?

Aries is not all that content when he is alone. So when he masturbates, he uses pornography both to turn him on and keep him company.

"It has a place for me in terms of personal stimulation."

"I love pornography and the strange thing is that I prefer straight porn to gay porn."

"I enjoy it as an art form. It is great entertainment but some of it is too graphic for me to enjoy."

HOW MUCH CUDDLING DO YOU ENJOY, ASIDE FROM SEX?

Aries loves feeling close to his lover. It is important to him to be touched, to be hugged, in the course of a day.

"I would prefer to cuddle over having sex."

"I am a very affectionate person and crave affection all the time."

"I love cuddling as much as sex."

FANTASIES

"I have fantasized about experimenting with a woman, because I like watching straight pornography. I don't think I really want to, but there is an awful turn-on with those videos. Maybe if there were two men and a woman it would be a possibility."

"I am at a balmy island at a nudist camp among a group of hunky men of various ages. What follows next is lots of foreplay and group sex, daily . . ."

A MEMORY

"I was having an argument with an ex-boyfriend and he shoved me. I pushed him against the wall, pinning him there. We were both turned-on. We began wrestling. I pinned him again and bit him. He got off right away. I got what I needed, then we went for a run through the woods and repeated it all there."

HOW TACTILE AND HOW ORAL ARE YOU?

He is quite tactile but even more oral. Kisses are important and Aries really appreciates a man who puts a lot of feeling into kissing him.

"I am extremely tactile, constantly touching, feeling, grabbing."

"I love deep kissing and fellatio, kissing all over except rimming."

"A little kissing on the mouth, they have to be really good. I love rolling my tongue over their hard sweaty body and biting his nipples, but no rimming."

WHAT SEX ACTS DO YOU LIKE MOST AND LEAST?

He is quite experimental in his range of sexual practices and finds little to dislike about sex, except that he isn't likely to use toys that may be painful, such as body clips, and he seldom participates in bondage.

"I love oral sex, mutual masturbation, having my balls licked, being fucked 'til orgasm, and I'll please him any way he wants."

"I like getting screwed. Actually it needs to be done right, slow, until you are ready, then steady."

"I used to love anal sex, but I stopped in the age of AIDS. Doing it was okay, but I really enjoyed getting it, especially if I had a hairy man on top of me. I would come to orgasm, masturbating myself, while he was performing anal sex. Now it is a fantasy for me."

"Can't think of anything I dislike with a man."

AS A LOVER, WHAT'S YOUR BEST SKILL?

Aries is particularly skilled at kissing and performing oral sex.

"I am a very slow rhythmic lover, my tongue is my best asset."

"I love kissing all over his hard sweaty body, fellatio, moving my tongue into all those tight small spots, and moving my fingertips everywhere, nice and light."

WHAT SMELLS AND TASTES ON YOUR PARTNER DO YOU ENJOY?

His partner's scents turn him on. Colognes might not. He loves the taste of skin and fresh sweat on a clean body.

"I don't like fragrance or dirt. I like the smell of a clean body, but sweat, that's okay, like someone who's just been to the gym. That can be pretty hot."

"I enjoy cologne, skin, and manly funky odors like armpits and crotch smells."

"I enjoy the smell of his testosterone, natural musk, underarms, and hair on his head."

"Taste of smooth skin, moist lips, a clean ass hole."

FOR SOME PEOPLE THE TASTE OF THEIR PARTNER'S CUM IS UNPLEASANT. IF THAT'S TRUE FOR YOU, HOW DO YOU HANDLE IT?

He doesn't enjoy the taste of cum and tries to avoid taking it into his mouth.

"I spit it out."

"I rub it on myself as a masturbation lubricant."

"I don't usually taste it. It's tacky, sweet . . . It tastes and smells like Clorox."

"I try to deal with it. It's not a pleasant moment."

"I do not swallow or rub it. I use a towel to wipe it up or roll around with it still on our bodies for a bit."

DO YOU ENJOY WATCHING YOUR PARTNER DURING SEX AND ORGASM? DO YOU ENJOY BEING WATCHED?

As a child taking chances, climbing that tall tree, learning to ride his bike, he wanted to be sure Mommy was nearby but not watching too protectively. After all, Aries sees himself as very independent. His behavior in this area is similar. He likes to look and see what his partner is doing but isn't all that comfortable if his lover observes him too closely.

"It is a turn on to watch what someone is doing to himself, to look at his body."

"Yes, I enjoy it when they orgasm. It gets me off."

"How I feel about being watched depends on the circumstances."

"I'm not really comfortable when I know he is looking at me."

The Big "O"

A MEMORY

"My first gay encounter. I was in my late teens. He was a good ten years older. We went into a small den. In minutes we had our clothes off and were on the floor. I wasn't sure what to do but I'd read stuff and knew that you'd engage in certain activities, mostly sucking someone's dick. So I did. In a few minutes it was over and off I went. I thought, 'I liked this, I'd like to come back.' And I did, once more."

HOW DO YOU REACH AN ORGASM AND HOW OFTEN?

Aries reaches orgasm virtually every time he has sex via masturbation and by a combination of other sex acts.

"It's easy for me to reach orgasm, usually through masturbation."

"I climax with oral sex to masturbation or sometimes when I am being fucked."

"I seldom reach orgasm unless I masturbate."

WHAT'S YOUR FAVORITE POSITION?

His preference is to be on top regardless of the exact nature of the position.

"I am usually straddling him, on my knees, sitting over his face. He likes rimming and stroking me at the same time. He prefers masturbating himself, so when he is getting close, I say 'Okay, give me my dick back' and then I play catch up."

"I like to be on top with him pinned beneath me."

"I'm on top of a guy with his legs over my shoulders, jerking him off."

SOME PEOPLE ARE CONCERNED ABOUT BRINGING A PARTNER TO CLIMAX BEFORE HAVING AN ORGASM THEMSELVES. OTHERS STRIVE TO REACH ORGASM TOGETHER. WHICH IS TRUE FOR YOU?

Aries is the "me first" sign of the zodiac, but when it comes to orgasm, he says sequence doesn't matter. Cumming together is desirable but that's not usually an objective.

"We were supposed to be studying, but ended up making love. We came at the same time. It was like magic. Afterwards, we just held each other."

"I would prefer mutual orgasm, but it doesn't happen often. I am usually first."

"With my partner we are pretty in sync and try to reach orgasm together."

"Orgasm together is best. If not, then them first."

ARE YOU VOCAL DURING SEX?

Relating to the way that he communicates his sexual likes and dislikes, he is more physical than verbal. He makes low moans rather than speaking to show his pleasure.

AFTER SEX WHAT DO YOU LIKE TO DO?

Aries doesn't want to do anything particularly active after sex.

"I like to sleep or talk and then relax with a movie."

"The best is just enjoying quiet moments. I don't want to do much."

"Rest, sometimes take a shower before curling up to sleep."

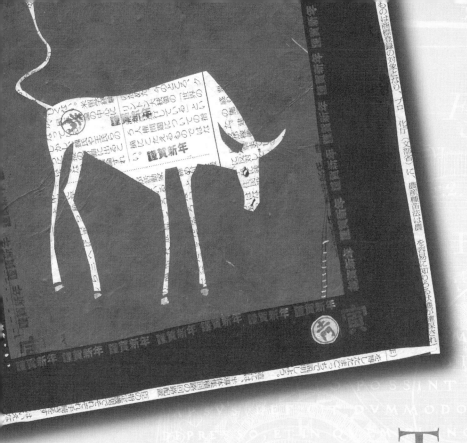

Taurus
THE BULL
April 20 through May 20

EARTH SIGN TAURUS, loyal, dependable, passionate, and highly physical, wants to move slowly and luxuriate in a backrub or full body massage. The Sign of Taurus rules the throat and the neck, the tongue, and the sense of touch. Taurus lovers have exceptionally sensitive hands.

What he says: "I do love to touch people in a sensual way. I could spend hours kissing someone who really does it well. I love to lick all over, especially arm pits, anus, scrotum, penis, belly, tits, everywhere."

"Let's get physical, physical . . . let me hear your body talk."

—Olivia Newton John

The Taurus Man
in His Own Words

"We were in a bright, airy room. There were large windows, the drapes were moving in the wind. I remember that we were lying in a luxurious bed, my lover kissed me all over, licked me, touched me, looked into my eyes and said 'I am yours.' He put lube on his dick and entered me slowly. I went crazy, screamed and begged him to go deeper. I remember the smell of his sweat, the drops of sweat falling on my face and pinching his nipples until I made him cum."

Attraction and Dating a Taurus

WHAT ATTRACTS YOU TO SOMEONE?

Taurus is the Sign of touch. He is a very physical man, sometimes mistaking lust for love. Good looks are tremendously important to him and on the subject of size, he may say it doesn't matter. In truth, he prefers a man with a large penis.

"Good hygiene matters and nice penis size, but what's most important of all is the ability to connect emotionally and spiritually with me."

"I am attracted by an air of confidence, a seriousness, a sense that someone is rather private. I appreciate a man who is devoted to his loved ones and also has a sense of humor."

"I'm a bit of a size queen and I like a man with strong chiseled features, an awesome sense of humor, and someone who is outgoing and caring."

WHAT MIGHT TURN YOU OFF?

If a man is out of shape and takes poor care of himself, Taurus is unlikely to be attracted. In addition, men who are narrow-minded turn him off.

"I am turned off by the typical things like being overweight, having poor hygiene or bad teeth, bad manners, and also being too effeminate."

"Thin people do not do it for me. I like flesh."

WHAT DO YOU ENJOY DOING ON A DATE?

Taurus might like seeing a movie, going to the theater, taking a walk, or having a wonderful conversation. But whatever else, one element is indispensable: food. Whether dining out, cooking together, or shopping at the supermarket, sharing food should be part of the evening. Sex will be dessert.

"Dinner always, sometimes walking around the city, and then having sex."

"Drinks, dinner, theater, and home for sex."

FANTASIES

"Being naked at home and having a UPS driver or a door-to-door missionary come to my house. We start doing it right then and there in the front hall."

"A threesome with me in the middle of two guys, one anal behind me, fucking me, and me anally fucking the guy in front—man sandwich."

ARE YOU FLIRTATIOUS?

He has an easygoing nature that attracts others to him. Even if he feels a bit insecure, he comes across as friendly and accessible.

"I am very flirtatious, live for flirting."

"Very, very much, babies, old ladies, hot guys, girls."

"Yes. Do what I can to get someone's attention."

ARE YOU JEALOUS?

Perhaps jealous is the wrong word for Taurus. He is possessive, about everything, and that certainly includes the man who is his lover.

"I can be jealous of people who have what I want."

"I would say I am fairly jealous."

"I have had my jealous moments and I am not proud of it."

HOW DO YOU FEEL ABOUT PUBLIC DISPLAYS OF AFFECTION?

Taurus loves to touch, so holding hands and other subtle displays that reinforce his connection to his partner are welcome.

"Holding hands, walking arm in arm, hugging, kissing is good. Making out is bad."

"Nothing heavy. Hugs and kisses are fine and only in gay-friendly places."

"Little ones like handholding are fine. Sucking tongues in the middle of the street is too much."

Sexual Attitudes and Behaviors

• •

HOW OFTEN DO YOU THINK ABOUT SEX AND HOW OFTEN PER WEEK DO YOU WANT TO HAVE SEX?

Any good-looking man walking by, any romantic setting or song on the radio will turn his thoughts to sex.

"I am thinking about it right now. I think about it often."

"I think about sex daily, numerous times daily . . . hourly."

He'd like to have sex more often, but three or four times a week will suffice.

"Sex every day, please."

"Almost every day."

"I want to have sex every other day when I am in a relationship."

MEMORIES

"One with a straight, hot-looking guy, because it had seemed so forbidden. He had just gotten engaged. Another, with a marine, which was just pure lust. I had known him for some time before the encounter, and it culminated in the first and only time I allowed myself to be fucked."

"I was with this great looking guy. He had a fantastic body and was also smart and sweet. It was the first time I did not consciously think about my performance. Rather I let myself completely drown in the warmth of his body, the taste and smell of his skin and his tongue and his cum and the thunderous rumblings of his groans of pleasure."

A MEMORY

"I was at the baths in New York City, sucking a guy's cock and balls. He was lying on his back and I was on my knees. First one guy came up from behind and fucked me, then a second, and then a third. After the third guy climaxed, he kissed me on the cheek. I was pleasantly surprised to see that it was my partner."

HOW LONG DO YOU LIKE TO SPEND HAVING SEX AND HOW MUCH OF THAT TIME IS FOREPLAY? DO YOU ENJOY QUICKIES?

Taurus likes thirty minutes to an hour, including lots of teasing and foreplay. Quickies are only okay, not terribly satisfying, and best as a prelude to longer sessions.

"One hour, quickies no."

"I don't enjoy quickies. I like taking my time including perhaps more foreplay than most people want."

"Sometimes the entire encounter is just foreplay, with no orgasm. If the person is right then I don't need to ejaculate, my brain already has."

WHAT TIME OF DAY DO YOU PREFER TO HAVE SEX?

Morning is fine. Evening is good. There's nothing wrong with night either. Taurus enjoys sex anytime.

"I enjoy sex at night, though whenever else is good too."

"Morning is best, I think. It sets the tone for the whole day."

"The morning is my favorite . . . late night too."

"Anytime can work, although we seem to really enjoy it when we are already late for something."

HOW OFTEN PER WEEK DO YOU MASTURBATE?

He goes through periods when he masturbates every day. Otherwise he does so three times a week.

HOW LONG DO YOU WANT TO KNOW SOMEONE BEFORE GETTING SEXUAL?

For anonymous sex he makes a quick judgment. When he meets a man who intrigues him and he anticipates a more serious relationship, he's likely to wait a week or so.

"The more I really like someone, the longer I delay getting into a physical relationship."

"I am up for sex as soon as the attraction is present."

"I don't have to know a man at all. If they are my type physically, I'm on my knees."

WHAT'S YOUR ATTITUDE TOWARD CASUAL SEX?

Taurus loves casual sex for the sheer physicality, the release. He strives to practice it safely.

"I love it. If there were no health risks, I would never hesitate. Morally I am fine with it."

"I'm single, I'm allowed."

"Love it. It's just a fun sport, not an emotional involvement."

DO YOU BELIEVE IN MONOGAMY?

Dating is one thing, commitment is another. Taurus is a Sign noted for loyalty. Monogamy is fundamental for him in order to feel stable and secure in a relationship.

"Nothing is better than being so into someone that there's no place you'd rather be than with him."

"Yes, if I'm in a relationship. If I'm just dating, anything goes."

"I'm in a 'don't ask, don't tell' relationship but I aspire to complete monogamy."

DOES SEX HAVE A SPIRITUAL SIGNIFICANCE FOR YOU?

Absolutely, aside from casual sex, intimacy transcends the physical plane.

"Definitely. Sex is magic when performed with someone you love. I pray that someone will come into my life whom I can love that much."

"It does when I am with someone I find physically and mentally compatible."

"Sex unites people on a deeper level than the everyday."

"It is a connection between my soul and the ability to give myself to a loved one."

ARE YOU COMFORTABLE INITIATING SEXUAL ACTIVITIES?

Taurus is so into touch, so much of a physical person, he has no trouble giving signals of his interest. Unless the message he gets back is a firm denial, he will continue to hint. Even in a totally new situation, if the other is encouraging, Taurus will initiate.

"Yes, I'm fine with opening the conversation or making the first moves, but I enjoy someone else initiating too."

A MEMORY

"My most romantic moments have not included sex at all, just cuddling or being close with someone. Sexually my favorite moments are the ones where my partner was very verbal, letting me know just what he liked and didn't like, and praising me when I found just the right spot."

HOW DO YOU COMMUNICATE TO YOUR PARTNER YOUR SEXUAL WANTS AND NEEDS?

Taurus may not always be the most talkative person, but when it comes to sex he is pretty direct and comfortable letting his partner know what is working and what isn't.

"I use verbal and non-verbal cues, but once we know each other well, gestures will do it."

"Like to talk about it beforehand to make sure that we have the same kinky interests."

DO YOU THINK OF YOURSELF AS BEING IN THE MAINSTREAM SEXUALLY, MORE EXPERIMENTAL, OR OPEN TO ANYTHING?

Taurus is a primarily mainstream lover, whose range of sexual activities includes kissing, oral and anal sex. The more experimental Tauran will try sex in public places, ménage à trois, spanking, and will occasionally incorporate food and dildoes into his sexual play. The most open of Tauran lovers is into water sports.

"I am done experimenting. I have tried leather, bondage, water sports, scat, public sex, group sex, rubber, anonymous sex, S&M, now I prefer just sucking and fucking."

His sexual fantasies involve anonymous sex, being with heterosexual men, or encounters with multiple partners.

HOW DO YOU DEMONSTRATE AFFECTION FOR YOUR PARTNER?

Taurus is loyal, loving, and thoughtful to his partner. He is helpful and supportive and shows his regard by preparing food.

"Many ways, baking cookies, cards, touches, hugs, loving words."

"Cooking dinner, telling him how I feel, and paying less attention to others."

"If I am in love with someone I will do his laundry, cook for him, and give lots of hugs and kisses."

"Getting involved in what he enjoys, preparing breakfast, being there for him."

The Five Senses

HOW IMPORTANT TO YOU IS THE SEXUAL ENVIRONMENT?

Venus, the planet of love and luxury, rules the Sign of Taurus. Therefore, a comfortable warm setting with sensual lighting, and perhaps soft music, all make the sexual experience richer for Taurus.

"Temperature and humidity are extremely important. Too cold or too hot doesn't work. Lighting should be dim. Other than that, anything works."

"I prefer clean, but I like manly smells a lot, sweat and piss, and there must be the right lighting."

"I enjoy a clean, neat environment, nice candle scents, incense, and music."

FANTASIES

"I like to fantasize about boys in their late teens and early twenties becoming my sex slaves."

"I fantasize being tied down by a hot man and forced to take him in my mouth and asked if I am enjoying it."

"Directing my own porno film, meeting the best looking man in the room, then going home with him for sex."

"I fantasize about being used as a sex toy with multiple partners and with my partner in charge. I am often handcuffed."

"I dream of kneeling on the floor while I suck off a line of young men. They all cum on my face."

A MEMORY

"I met a man in Thailand. We went to a bathhouse . . . it was warm, humid. We were in a small room that was made especially for sex. This was our first of many encounters. We were so in tune with each other that the experience felt more like a synchronized dance than sex. When I moved, he moved at the same time in exactly the right way. Maybe it was just being so far from home, that I was able to relax and let my guard down, without having to worry about who I am supposed to be."

WHERE DO YOU LIKE TO HAVE SEX?

Given the fact that Taurus loves creature comforts, being warm, lying on soft pillows, the bedroom is his favorite place to have sex. On rare occasions, he is open to having sex in unexpected settings, but he would prefer to postpone it long enough to get home.

"The conventional bedroom is best but I wouldn't be averse to trying something different."

"In private, beds mostly, sometimes in the woods, and a car is particularly exciting."

"Warm dark places where no one else can see."

"Any place I can get away with it without being arrested. I love public sex. I once had sex on a train platform."

WHAT PUTS YOU IN THE MOOD FOR SEX?

Start with food. Go out to dinner or share a home cooked meal, take out Chinese, even head to the supermarket. He has a sensual nature and food puts him in the mood.

"Warm and cozy atmosphere, logs burning in the fireplace, low lights."

"Music is a must, cleanliness is a must, ambiance is just window dressing. The right guy will always get me in the mood."

"If the time and the person is right, I need nothing to stimulate me."

"The environment can do it, such as being in the woods or a really comfortable spot. The aroma of the person I am with can definitely do it, as long as it is not perfume. It has to be his own scent."

WHAT'S YOUR ATTITUDE TOWARD PORNOGRAPHY?

Taurus has a love/hate relationship with pornography. He admits that it turns him on, but he may be uncomfortable with it for varying reasons. Poorly done porn only makes him feel more alone.

"It is alluring, yet somewhat repulsive."

"It's okay now and then. I find when I am lonely it makes those feeling worse."

"Love it/hate it. It is good for five minutes then I am turned off. It makes me feel a little dirty, sacrilegious, if that makes sense."

"I like it only for masturbation purposes, not when I am playing with someone."

"It is okay if it turns the other person on. I have very little interest in it."

HOW MUCH CUDDLING DO YOU ENJOY, ASIDE FROM SEX?

Taurus is a highly physical Sign and uses touch to communicate his connection to a person, to signal interest in sex, or just to be comforting.

"I think cuddling is the key to making the connection, to opening the door to good sex."

"I am a very affectionate person, so if I like someone I am very touchy-feely."

"I love to cuddle, I am a touchy-feely, kind of guy, very romantic and affectionate."

HOW TACTILE ARE YOU AND HOW ORAL ARE YOU?

Taurus is very oral, but even more tactile. He loves to move his hands all over his partner's body, sometimes closing his eyes and losing himself in the sense of touch.

"Touching really turns me on. I am very tactile."

"I love to feel smooth skin all over. I will lick and suck any clean body part."

"I am very oral if the person is clean. I love to kiss all over his body."

"I like to give oral sex, love to get rimmed."

"I could rub someone all day. I do love to touch people in a sensual way. I could spend hours kissing someone who really does it well. I love to lick all over, especially arm pits, anus, scrotum, penis, belly, tits, everywhere."

> ### FANTASIES
>
> "I love imagining that I'm wrestling, nude or in Speedos or Lycra."
>
> "Being gang banged. An orgy atmosphere, in a college locker room with a bunch of jocks, steamy, sweaty."
>
> "I am smitten with this guy who is twenty and apparently straight. I have often wished he would fall for me, marry me, and we would live happily ever after. And then I run into him and he welcomes my advances."

A FANTASY

"I am in a men's room that has hundreds of stalls. There is no roof on this facility; it is open to the air and sky. I go from stall to stall pleasuring each man, as all of them want me badly. One after another cries out in pleasure as I am touching him. And I enjoy each and every one. The love I give out and receive is palpable; in fact, the sexual energy creates a buzzing sound, like electricity gaining momentum. The dream is never quite long enough."

WHAT SEX ACTS DO YOU LIKE MOST AND LEAST?

As he is a primarily mainstream lover, his range of sex acts includes kissing, oral sex, fondling, and anal sex, pretty much in that order. He doesn't much enjoy mutual masturbation or nipple play and he is not interested in BDSM sex toys such as body clips, paddles, or restraints. A gentle spanking, however, when he is a "bad boy" is definitely deserved.

"I do not enjoy anything that involves extraneous props."

"I love kissing, oral sex, sucking dick, balls, and ass, ass play, and fucking, both giving and receiving."

"Anything as long as it involves mutual pleasure. Kissing is high on my list. I don't like pain or constriction, just two or more bodies entwined."

AS A LOVER, WHAT'S YOUR BEST SKILL?

He is a good lover generally because he has a caring nature and he is a master at thrilling a lover with the use of his mouth and tongue.

"My tongue talks volumes all over their bodies."

"Kissing and licking, rimming and sucking."

"I am a deeply passionate, strong lover, attentive to my lover's needs. I am equally anxious to please him as well as myself."

"I am about the best rimmer ever born."

WHAT SMELLS AND TASTES ON YOUR PARTNER DO YOU ENJOY?

Taurus is a very sensual Sign. His partner's natural body smells are appealing to him. He also likes the saltiness of a little sweat and if he uses food, his preference is for something sweet, like honey.

"I enjoy every clean smell, his penis and scrotum, as well as every taste."

"For smells, natural body odors, ball sack, underarm, ass, hair on head. For tastes, the sweetness of a wet kiss and tasting myself on him."

"I enjoy the smell of his skin, colognes, and the taste of chocolate pudding and whipped cream on his skin."

"I don't like cologne, perfume, deodorant, or any other man-made chemical. I love the smell of armpits, clean or not, scrotums, clean or not. Butt holes, clean or not more than a day old. And definitely his dirty underpants, oh yes I like those."

FOR SOME PEOPLE THE TASTE OF THEIR PARTNER'S CUM IS UNPLEASANT. IF THAT'S TRUE FOR YOU, WHAT DO YOU DO ABOUT THE TASTE?

Taurus seldom has any problem with the tastes of cum, but even if he does, as he wants to please his partner, he willingly swallows it.

"I love the taste of my partner's cum. I would rather swallow it than see it go to waste."

"I love cum in my mouth or on my face."

"I could eat cum all day and love having it sprayed all over my chest or anywhere it lands."

A MEMORY

"It was near closing time at the convenience store that I went into frequently. The young manager was there alone and asked me to stick around. He took me into the back room and told me how he couldn't hide his desire for me any more and pulled me in close. His eyes were big and expressive and he had crazy hair. He kissed me gently, cautiously, then deeper, opened my shirt and kissed my chest, down to my cock. Then he proceeded to make love to my dick and loved it because it was me. And at that moment he relinquished himself to me."

DO YOU ENJOY WATCHING YOUR PARTNER DURING SEX AND ORGASM? DO YOU ENJOY BEING WATCHED?

Taurus loves to observe the effect his lovemaking is having upon his partner and finds watching him a huge turn on. In spite of that, he is uncomfortable when he becomes aware that his partner is studying him.

"I like to look in someone's eyes when I am going down on him."

The Big "O"

A FANTASY

"A surprise visit from someone with whom I haven't yet been sexual. He is very masculine, but I am able to turn him into my bitch. I put him on his knees while he is doing me. I imagine him looking up at me while sucking my dick, then flipping him over, or raising his legs, and rimming him until I know he is ready and having him say 'Please fuck me,' and moaning when I do. Perfect."

A FANTASY

"69ing with a hot man . . . anonymous encounters with extremely sexy men—Colt Men. I like to fantasize about young men, say in their early twenties, becoming my sex slaves. In others I fantasize about hot sex, mainly with straight men and having outdoor sex, public or private sex, participating in an orgy."

HOW DO YOU REACH AN ORGASM AND HOW OFTEN?

He always achieves orgasm through masturbation, but may have difficulty reaching it by other means.

"Usually with a combination or getting a blow job along with anal sex or mutual masturbation."

"I only reach orgasm when I masturbate."

"If I am extremely excited all you have to do is touch my scrotum and I am off. When I ejaculate I am usually alone and masturbate with my finger firmly planted in my anus."

WHAT'S YOUR FAVORITE POSITION?

Facing side by side is the most common position for him but he also enjoys variety.

"Doggie style has been the most successful, but stomach to stomach is pretty hot."

"I like being on my back, with my partner above me in a 69 position."

SOME PEOPLE ARE CONCERNED ABOUT BRINGING A PARTNER TO CLIMAX BEFORE HAVING AN ORGASM THEMSELVES. OTHERS STRIVE TO REACH ORGASM TOGETHER. WHICH IS TRUE FOR YOU?

He loves achieving climax simultaneously but pleasing his partner is even more important.

"Usually my concern is to get the other person off. I truly enjoy bringing that pleasure to someone."

"Mutual orgasm is desirable, most of the time I tend to cum very quickly."

ARE YOU VOCAL DURING SEX?

He ranges from moderate to quite vocal during sex and orgasm.

"I am very vocal, as long as I am getting pleasure."

"With the right person I love to be vocal. It keeps me focused and aroused."

"I will moan rather than talk."

AFTER SEX WHAT DO YOU LIKE TO DO?

He wants to cuddle, relax, talk a little, and perhaps take a shower and sleep. Generally he prefers staying home after sex.

"I am a man, sleep, of course."

"Anything, everything, nothing."

"I usually sleep for a bit, then make breakfast, or go out for something to eat."

A FANTASY

"Sometimes I think about guys who I had sex with many years ago. I wonder how they would act if they come back, after a long time has gone by. I imagine them getting turned on, not telling me that they want to get screwed, but somehow making it clear that they really, really do. Another fantasy, straight guys, or those who think they are, being very coy when they need to be treated like a woman. Imagining their body language and the way they make the first move is very hot for me."

A MEMORY

"He walked in and said that I could do anything I wanted to him. He trusted me. He was a virgin and wanted to experience sex. He was clean, spotless. He spoke very little. It was quiet. He never said 'stop' to anything and it was wonderful."

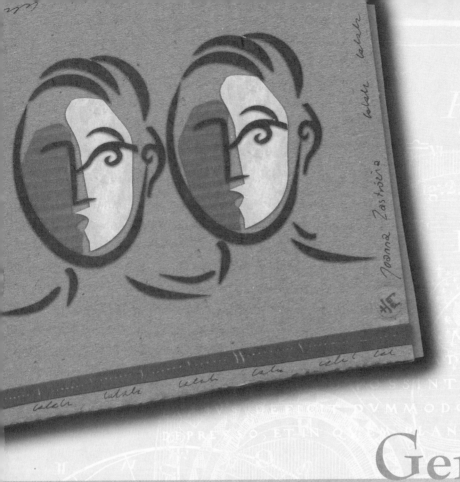

Gemini

THE TWINS

May 21 through June 20

"Love is the wind, the tide,

the waves, the sunshine."

—Henry David Thoreau,
"Paradise (To Be) Regained"

AIR SIGN GEMINI is into experimentation in all things from types of food to sexual behaviors. Ruler of the shoulders, arms, hands, and the sense of hearing, Gemini is turned on by all things auditory—the sounds of nature, music, and sexy talk.

What he says: "Before getting sexual I would like to know a man at least long enough to have some conversation and find out if he's more than a cock and an ass. Then, if the chemistry is good, go for it."

The Gemini Man in His Own Words

"A friend came over to do some work for me. He was wearing coveralls that zipped down the front. He got hot and sweaty and unzipped the coveralls down to his waist. He had nothing on underneath. His black pubic hairs were showing. Then he zipped down all the way and hung his balls and big hard cock out. Of course I had to help him get off, so he could get it back in his coveralls. He stood on a ladder so that his cock was right in my face. I love sucking."

Attraction and Dating a Gemini

WHAT ATTRACTS YOU TO SOMEONE?

Attracting Gemini's attention in the first place is almost purely physical but he is a man of broad interests, so holding his attention requires a complex personality and a curiosity about a range of topics.

"The first things I notice are a man's physique, weight, his hair, energy, and behavior. I am attracted by a man with strong muscles, good legs, and a nice butt."

"Uniforms are a big turn-on for me as well as a man in a suit."

"Face, eyes, lips to make me want to kiss him all the time."

"Confidence without egotism, smile, sense of humor."

"Physical characteristics catch my attention first, but then, intelligence, class, humor, compassion for the long-term. Let's face it, a pretty face will only go so far."

WHAT MIGHT TURN YOU OFF?

Turn-offs for him include lack of style, obesity, and smoking. He's also very independent and won't tolerate a possessive or clingy partner. Overall, a gorgeous man who can't carry on a conversation and has little interest in the world around him won't hold Gemini's interest for any length of time. The sex might be great, but there won't be a relationship. Arrogance is a turn-off quality on every Gemini's list.

"A person who doesn't take care of his body and is full of himself."

"Grossly overweight, better-than-thou attitude."

"Bad breath and teeth odor, arrogant attitude."

"Someone who thinks he is God's gift definitely turns me off."

A MEMORY

"I have a memory that is much more amusing than romantic. A gay friend of mine was going out with a very nice guy who was quite effeminate. That guy decided he wanted to have sex with me. We went to his place and started kissing and touching and all was going great until we took our clothes off. I was really surprised to find that he had an exceptionally tiny penis. I mean, it was hardly bigger than a woman's clitoris. I was so shocked that I lost my hard-on. I was expecting a guy and he was almost a girl."

WHAT DO YOU ENJOY DOING ON A DATE?

Gemini doesn't want to do anything particularly out of the ordinary on a date. He loves music and conversation, so an ideal evening might incorporate a concert and a quiet dinner for two or with a small group of close friends.

"Most of all I want to have fun, have something to eat and drink and especially share good conversation. If it leads to anything then so be it."

"In seducing or being seduced I like conversation, soft music, good food."

"Going out to dinner, movie, exploring new places, taking walks, sitting in a café and talking."

ARE YOU FLIRTATIOUS?

With his gregarious nature and easy ability to talk with anyone, he comes across as decidedly flirtatious. In his own opinion, there is no intention to be anything but friendly.

"I flirt every chance I get, whenever I feel any sort of bond."

"Yes, by winking, smiling, and constant staring."

"Loads, too much, so I am told."

ARE YOU JEALOUS?

His answer to this question is sort of "Yes, No, Maybe so." In fact he is a nervous type and apt to become edgy if he sees his partner flirting with other men.

"Yes, often but not too bad."

"No not really, well, just a little."

"When I was younger I used to be. Now I am more trusting and self-confident."

"Not by nature, just by instinct."

HOW DO YOU FEEL ABOUT PUBLIC DISPLAYS OF AFFECTION?

He enjoys observing other men displaying affection openly. However, his edgy disposition prevents him from engaging in more than minimal physical contact.

"A hug, a slight touch, a smile, a wink, the rest is private."

"I love them within gay settings."

"In most places it is great. Sometimes an environment just feels wrong."

"I feel warmed all over when I observe two men publicly showing affection for each other."

> ### FANTASIES
>
> "I would love to have a three-some where my partner is the watcher and then he can join in when I am reaching my orgasm . . . or having one huge orgy with lots of hot, young, muscular lean men who have tons of energy."
>
> "Being gang fucked, sucking a guy while getting fucked, 69 with a guy while getting fucked."

Sexual Attitudes and Behaviors

HOW OFTEN DO YOU THINK ABOUT SEX AND HOW OFTEN PER WEEK DO YOU WANT TO HAVE SEX?

Gemini is a very sexual Sign. He thinks about sex daily, if not hourly, and would like to have sex five times weekly.

HOW LONG DO YOU LIKE TO SPEND HAVING SEX AND HOW MUCH OF THAT TIME IS FOREPLAY? DO YOU ENJOY QUICKIES?

He likes to spend an hour having sex and has mixed feelings about quickies. He loves foreplay, "tons of foreplay . . . as long as it can last."

"I like to have one hour, sometimes longer, for a scene. Quickies are okay sometimes."

"I don't like quickies. I prefer long pleasurable sex."

"I like long passionate sex, hate quickies."

"Sometimes I like to spend a long time with someone I love, but I also enjoy a quickie on occasion."

"If it's a quickie with someone anonymous, then there is almost no foreplay. With a lover, the foreplay might go on for almost an hour."

FANTASIES

"My image is being caught masturbating by a man that gets turned on and who then thrills me by joining in. Other fantasies, group sex in a prison or locker room."

"Meeting a police officer or a fireman . . . being taken back to the station, firehouse, and fondled and handcuffed. Sitting in the fire engine, and just being touched and kissed all over, then having hot sweaty sex."

WHAT TIME OF DAY DO YOU PREFER TO HAVE SEX?

Gemini, with sex on his mind so much of the time, isn't overly fussy about time of day for sex. If he has any preference, it's in the morning before the day gets busy.

"Time of day doesn't really matter, but sex in the morning is really great."

"My preference is before or after sleep, if it is a loving relationship. For casual sex, any time will do."

HOW OFTEN DO YOU MASTURBATE?

He averages four times per week.

HOW LONG DO YOU WANT TO KNOW SOMEONE BEFORE GETTING SEXUAL?

No question about it, if he finds a man physically attractive, he'll be feeling ready. But, in fact, he wants to talk with a man long enough to add another dimension before becoming sexually involved.

"Ideally, I'd like to know someone a few months or at least three or four dates before getting sexual. In reality, I usually get sexual before I know the person at all well."

"This depends on the person. It could be five minutes, could be months."

"More than a day."

"Before getting sexual I would like to know a man at least long enough to have some conversation and find out if he's more than a cock and an ass. Then, if the chemistry is good, go for it."

"When it is right it can be anytime."

"There is no need for a waiting period. Mutual desire is all that is required."

WHAT'S YOUR ATTITUDE TOWARD CASUAL SEX?

He is a smart man and a nervous one who likes casual sex. As long as precautions are taken, he is open to it and to anonymous sex.

"I think of sex as part recreation, part sharing, part communication."

"Of course, precautions are necessary. If no condoms are used I think it is stupidly unsafe."

"It is fine, but I want more."

A MEMORY

"Met in a bar, in the bathroom actually, came out and got a drink and sat down next to him. We chatted for a while and started kissing. I went back to his hotel and we had oral sex, because we didn't have condoms with us. The next three days we just hung out and his last night in New York we debated for over an hour whether or not to have anal sex. We both had adoring boyfriends at home. After tears, we went back to his hotel and had sex. I put him on the airport bus, and have not seen or talked to him since. I miss and love him a lot. Those were the best four days of my life. Ultimately, I ended my eight-year relationship with my boyfriend. I let the love of my life go free."

DO YOU BELIEVE IN MONOGAMY?

Gemini has a nervous disposition and worries about trusting his partner. Being faithful, therefore, is very important to him and he believes in monogamy.

"Yes, however, I don't see it very often in the gay community."

"Yes. I believe a commitment with one person makes sex even more special."

"Yes, in a certain sense. My partner and I engage in sexual activities with other guys, but only when we are together. We have anal sex only with each other."

A MEMORY

"My lover and a good friend of ours spent the night at our summer home. I left written instructions for them, telling them that the following morning, at a certain hour, the friend was to be bent over a stool, with his ass up and lubed, while he sucked my lover, waiting for me to fuck him. I arrived after a five-hour trip and mounted the bottom, then my lover."

"I believe it is possible, but the chemistry has to be right."

DOES SEX HAVE A SPIRITUAL SIGNIFICANCE FOR YOU?

The sexual connection is so much more than just the physical for Gemini. It represents true intimacy.

"Anything that contributes to connection with another person may have a spiritual significance for me. That includes sharing food, conversation, and sex."

"With my life partner, yes. Sex with other people is just for the physical aspect."

"In terms of true intimacy, yes. Intimacy heightens my soul and intensifies the pleasurable satisfaction of sex."

ARE YOU COMFORTABLE INITIATING SEXUAL ACTIVITIES?

Given his somewhat nervous disposition and the fact that he is seldom aggressive or even pushy, Gemini needs some signal of interest from another man before he will initiate the idea of becoming sexual. Once the ground is broken, he's quite comfortable initiating sex.

"If there is some indication that the other person is open to such activities, then I am very comfortable being the initiator."

HOW DO YOU COMMUNICATE TO YOUR PARTNER YOUR SEXUAL WANTS AND NEEDS?

Gemini rules communication. He is good at getting his point across, and to indicate his desires, he uses a combination of words and gestures with slightly more emphasis on sounds.

"I usually try to reinforce what he does that pleases me by making audible sounds of pleasure. Sometimes I will also use words or gestures."

DO YOU THINK OF YOURSELF AS BEING IN THE MAINSTREAM SEXUALLY, MORE EXPERIMENTAL, OR OPEN TO ANYTHING?

Gemini is a pretty experimental lover. He is open to group sex, sex in public places, exhibitionism, voyeurism, using costumes including leather and latex, underwear, as well as spanking and bondage, and he loves playing with sex toys such as dildoes, vibrators. Some Geminis also use butt plugs, handcuffs cock rings, ball stretchers, and nipple clamps. He loves the "vacuum cleaner."

His fantasy life is an extension of his sexual behaviors.

HOW DO YOU DEMONSTRATE AFFECTION FOR YOUR PARTNER?

He will almost always help his partner when requested. He just might not know to offer. Gemini means to be attentive and caring but he is apt to forget the traditional occasions for gifts, like anniversaries. Truly he will appreciate being told what is desired and being given reminders of important dates.

FANTASIES

"Uniforms and a man in a suit are big turn-ons for me. I picture a guy letting me suck him the way I want to and then he does the same for me."

"I imagine myself in either of two extreme positions. I'm a dominant top or a submissive bottom. I am restrained and forced to cum or forced to perform oral sex. Sometimes I fantasize about the pleasure of being caught masturbating and the thrill of the person joining me."

"With hugs, holding hands, compliments, gently touching him a lot, looking in his eyes, fucking him tenderly."

"Making life as easy as possible in small and large ways."

"Buy flowers, write a note, or call to say 'hi,' cook dinner, meet for lunch and buy it."

"Listening to him, selfless acts, giving a good body massage, and telling him I love him."

"Verbal expressions are a biggy. Hugging and touching are important. Paying obvious attention to him is also very important."

The Five Senses

HOW IMPORTANT TO YOU IS THE SEXUAL ENVIRONMENT?

Remembering that Gemini has a nervous disposition, a primary concern for him, when it comes to the setting for sex, is that it be safe. Beyond that, he does appreciate cleanliness and candlelight.

"It should be dimly lit and clean, but not fastidiously so."

"Cleanliness is a must."

"I care about the décor, candles, and romance."

"It needs to be clean for sure."

A MEMORY

"I was living in New York City at the time, and went into a neighborhood bar. I noticed a good-looking older man who was talking with some friends. He had a marvelous voice. Later I found out he was a radio personality. We got to talking and he made it clear he wanted to have sex with me. We went to his apartment. It was a basement level two bedroom, quite plush. All he wanted was to give me a blow job. He didn't expect anything in return. Adding to the experience, he had a partner who was asleep in another room and who slept through our entire encounter."

WHERE DO YOU LIKE TO HAVE SEX?

He loves to have sex in a car. The Sign of Gemini rules automobiles. Sexy cars turn him on. He also enjoys watching what's going on and well-placed mirrors heighten his pleasure.

"I have not found a place where I do not like to have sex."

WHAT PUTS YOU IN THE MOOD FOR SEX?

Showering together is one guaranteed turn-on. The other is anything having to do with sexy cars. Parking in a quiet secluded place, illuminated only by the stars, puts him in the mood.

"Waking up with a hard-on, seeing or hearing other men having sex (in person or on video), looking over at my lover lying asleep, showering together, aromas, and music."

"Spending time together, showering, hanging out in the nude, inside or outside."

"Low lights, hot weather, sweaty men, pornography, low thumping tribal music."

"Sometimes I am physically horny and then I go looking for sex. At other times, a lover will initiate sex usually by touching me and I will quickly respond in kind."

WHAT'S YOUR ATTITUDE TOWARD PORNOGRAPHY?

Porn is okay for self-pleasure. It isn't that much of a turn on with a partner. His taste in porn leans toward mainstream sex, orgies, and mostly cum shots.

"I like it when all else fails."

"Porn is okay. I prefer the real experience."

"I think it is one of the delightful facets of sexual pleasure."

> ### A MEMORY
>
> "One summer night, I went camping and had sex under a beautiful moonlit sky. Every star in the universe was out. The smell of the woods, that range of natural outdoor aromas, made me so hot and horny while being fucked. The sounds of the crickets and an owl, which I swear hooted every time he thrust into me, made me go so wild that I had to orgasm before he came. He loved every minute of it, being his first time with someone like me with all this energy. Best weekend ever."

HOW MUCH CUDDLING DO YOU ENJOY, ASIDE FROM SEX?

He loves to touch and be touched, to kiss and cuddle. But most often the activity does lead to sex.

"I just love to cuddle with someone I love, however, I regard this as sexual, even if it is not oriented or directed to climax."

HOW TACTILE AND HOW ORAL ARE YOU?

Gemini rules the hands. He is wonderful at exciting his lover with his sense of touch. He is also highly oral but rimming is an activity reserved only for his monogamous partner.

"I have great hands and love to explore all his maleness, to give him a massage . . . it's all part of foreplay."

"Kissing, mouth and body. Yes! Yes! Yes!"

"I am both very tactile and oral. I love to explore with

> ### A FANTASY
>
> "I usually rerun the memory of a sexual encounter that was aborted. The seduction time is always more exciting to me than the time of climax. Seduction usually involves verbal innuendoes and suggestive gestures."

my wandering hands and kiss his mouth and body, occasional rimming and fellatio."

WHAT SEX ACTS DO YOU LIKE MOST AND LEAST?

While he is a pretty experimental lover, the sex acts that he participates in most commonly are kissing, oral sex, and mutual masturbation. Anal sex may or may not be to his liking. Either way, he is more apt to be top than bottom. He is rarely into heavy bondage or sadomasochism.

"I like for a guy to let me suck him the way I want to and then return the favor. I have fun sucking a flat stomach. I just love sucking a nice clean cock."

"I don't like getting fucked or him cumming in my mouth."

"Most of all I like to give oral pleasure while receiving hand manipulation of my penis."

A FANTASY

"In my mind I envision a man who is muscular, well built, not a body builder but very athletic, blond. He will let me do anything I want to him. I give him the best blow job he's ever had in his life and then he reciprocates."

AS A LOVER, WHAT'S YOUR BEST SKILL?

His willingness to experiment may be his greatest skill. He is proud of the use of his tongue but may underestimate how gifted he is with his hands.

"I am very oral. As a top I have great stamina and I cum with great force and distance."

"I think I am good at giving a blow job. I am also good at being an active participant while my lover fucks me."

"My hands and the way I give a massage. I've been told that I'm very skilled with my mouth and tongue."

WHAT SMELLS AND TASTES ON YOUR PARTNER DO YOU ENJOY?

Stick to clean smells to please him most. He prefers the taste of clean skin unadorned by colognes. He is comfortable with natural tastes, precum, and the crotch area, but there are no particular flavors that he likes on his partner. He isn't big on food mixed into the sexual experience.

"Favorite smells include soap, skin, and natural odors, cock, sweaty, musty, some ass scent."

"I don't like cologne. I don't mind his butt scent."

"I find myself gravitating to my partner's armpits. I can't perceive any smell but it does excite me."

"The sweetness of most precum is very pleasant."

FOR SOME PEOPLE THE TASTE OF THEIR PARTNER'S CUM IS UNPLEASANT. IF THAT'S TRUE FOR YOU, WHAT DO YOU DO ABOUT THE TASTE?

Gemini doesn't object to the taste, but he usually chooses to avoid cum with all except a committed partner. The Gemini who is in a monogamous relationship and doesn't adore the taste of his lover's cum keeps a bottle of mouthwash at the ready.

"I don't eat or taste cum. It is unsafe to do so and I wash it off my body immediately."

"It's been 15 years since I tasted cum, HIV worries ended that pleasure. Now I avoid getting it near my mouth, eyes, dick, or ass."

"I love the taste. It's not a problem."

"I worry about health issues so I prefer to not swallow cum."

FANTASIES

"My fantasies vary. Sometimes I am a dominant top and others I am a submissive bottom. I like to imagine being restrained and forced to cum."

"Fantasies for me include being teased or jacked off, a variety of normal and kink activities, also out of the ordinary locations with some sense of safe risk, parks, definitely the beach someday. Another fantasy is to give anal in a pool or in the ocean and last, having the sub get aggressive."

DO YOU ENJOY WATCHING YOUR PARTNER DURING SEX AND ORGASM? DO YOU ENJOY BEING WATCHED?

Gemini gets into the total experience of sex, relishing all senses. The experience of watching his lover as well as being watched in return adds another dimension to what he's feeling with his mouth and hands.

"When I get fucked I like using a mirror to watch my partner's penis go in and out. I just love cock."

A MEMORY

"I had been slightly flirting for quite some time with a maintenance man who worked for the same company that I did. We would exchange comments and looks in the halls and I knew that the attraction was mutual. One night he came into my office and proceeded to initiate some sexual activity by his conversation. We had quite a time of it, heightened by the danger of possibly being caught."

"Yes, I do. I also enjoy watching someone masturbate."

"I enjoy being an exhibitionist if it is evident that this is turning on the other person."

The Big "O"

HOW DO YOU REACH AN ORGASM AND HOW OFTEN?

Gemini has little trouble cumming. He needs variety and reaches orgasm by a combination of oral sex and masturbation and sometimes with anal sex.

"I usually reach orgasm by oral sex or hand manipulation."

"For me it's a combination, usually ending with me masturbating."

"Oral sex, masturbation, and combinations. I need variety."

WHAT'S YOUR FAVORITE POSITION?

He has some preference for doggie style and facing side by side, but there really isn't any one set position that he favors.

"I can achieve orgasm with my partner under me, doggie style, next to me, or facing side by side."

"Anything can happen, but I usually end up lying face down with my penis pulled back between my legs when I achieve orgasm."

SOME PEOPLE ARE CONCERNED ABOUT BRINGING A PARTNER TO CLIMAX BEFORE HAVING AN ORGASM THEMSELVES. OTHERS STRIVE TO REACH ORGASM TOGETHER. WHICH IS TRUE FOR YOU?

In most of the things that he does, Gemini manages to be both observer and participant at the same time. When having sex, this dual ability helps him to strive to reach orgasm simultaneously with his partner. He can hold back, watching for clues that his partner is about to cum, and then release himself at the same time.

"I prefer reaching simultaneous orgasms. It's not the focus, but it's nice when it happens."

"We try to achieve climax simultaneously, but it's not that important."

ARE YOU VOCAL DURING SEX?

Gemini is a verbal sign and can be fairly vocal during sex. He wants his partner to know what he's enjoying and appreciates hearing from his lover as well. His communication may be more sounds than words, but the meaning is clear.

"I am always at least a little vocal, sometimes very vocal."

"A lot, trust me."

"I'm very vocal during sex. Come on, I'm a Gemini."

MEMORIES

"It was a threesome, in my bedroom—highly erotic, sexually incredible."

"I met a guy at a bathhouse, very clean smells, very muscular guy, older, and more dominating."

AFTER SEX WHAT DO YOU LIKE TO DO?

After sex, he wants more sex. He'll want to stay up for a while afterward, watch a movie, talk quietly.

"I like to shower, have sex again, then eat something."

"Shower, go again, talk, and cuddle."

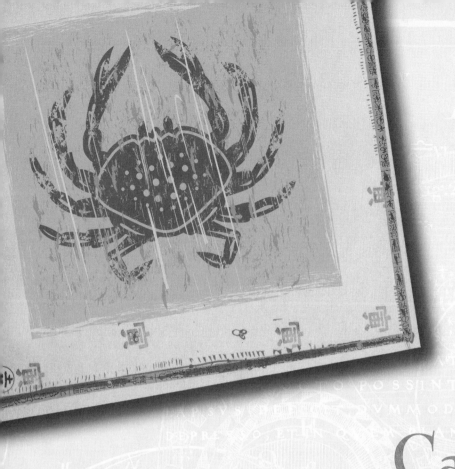

Cancer

THE CRAB

June 21 through July 22

WATER SIGN CANCER, nurturing and sensitive, is concerned with home, family, and food. Ruler of the breasts, stomach, and chest, Cancer is turned on by sharing food, emotional closeness, and feeling loved. Cancers like to have sex in the woods or by a body of water.

What he says: "How vocal I am during sex depends on the scene, usually lots of moans and slurps. I get very chatty and philosophical during sex, so sometimes you have to put something in my mouth to shut me up."

"As life's pleasures go,

food is second only to sex."

—Alan King

The Cancer Man in His Own Words

A MEMORY

"I met a guy cruising in the rambles in Central Park while I was visiting New York. The expression in his eyes and the smell of his cologne turned me on. We went to lunch, fed each other. Then on the street we held hands, kissed, frenched. At his apartment we had a few beers and listened to a tape of New Age music. We showered, kissing and touching, leading to more foreplay and anal sex with poppers and toys. Afterward, we went out dancing then returned to his place and I stayed over. In the morning he made breakfast and we fooled around again."

Attraction and Dating a Cancer

WHAT ATTRACTS YOU TO SOMEONE?

Cancer notices a man who appears relaxed, smiles, and is approachable. He cares that a man be in good physical shape and is attentive to his appearance. No specific physical attributes are of overriding importance. What matters more to him is that the man is close to his own family and will make an effort to relate well to Cancer's.

"I am attracted by a man's sense of humor and personality. Gentleness, vitality makes the person. Lack of it has made gorgeous people ugly to me. Deep blue eyes and muscular thighs are also appealing."

"Sense of humor, laugh, not overly muscular, animalistic sexual energy."

"What appeals to me is being well groomed and neatly dressed. I like steady eye contact, energy, and I notice a man's physique."

"How they move and hold themselves. Pecs are a real turn on. Mutual respect is required. Politeness is necessary."

WHAT MIGHT TURN YOU OFF?

Cancer is something of a homebody and is often a good cook. Perhaps that is why he focuses on a man's mouth. He is, therefore, turned off by someone who pays too little attention to his teeth or has bad breath. Cancer also has a nurturing quality and is best balanced by a man who is very masculine, therefore, a man who is overly feminine turns him off.

"Negative attitude or inappropriate language are barriers. On a first date he should be dressed neatly."

"When I meet a man who is arrogant, I'm not interested. Also bad style, poor teeth, and bad breath turn me off."

"Feminine behavior, vanilla, inexperience, bad health."

"Bad teeth, neurotic behavior, too femme."

"Feminine men."

FANTASIES

"A pirate scene, using leather and whips, using food. Most of all my fantasies involve sex on the beach, in a pool, or outside in the rain."

"I fantasize about sex in a group at a bath house or in the reeds or dunes of a beach."

"A hot jock in the locker room is getting ready to take a shower. He sees me watching him, comes over and says 'You want this hot body don't you?' I say 'Yes.' He brings me into the shower, tells me to suck his big manly cock. As I do it, he tells me how lucky I am to have him in my mouth."

WHAT DO YOU ENJOY DOING ON A DATE?

He is a Water Sign. Any date is enhanced if it is near water, the ocean, a pond, even poolside. Food is indispensable, home cooked or served at a restaurant, pizza or a sandwich in a quiet corner of the local pub.

"I enjoy anything as long as there is great conversation and great food."

"Laughing, talking about a common experience such as seeing a play or movie, eating delicious food and then having great sex."

"Having dinner and conversation, followed by sex, and then those quick good byes."

"Dinner out or in, walking, shopping, and sex."

ARE YOU FLIRTATIOUS?

Cancer has a remarkable ability to draw people out. Men and women alike are at ease talking with him. This quality amounts to a kind of comfortable flirtation.

"I flirt with everyone, male and female, gay and straight, because it's fun. Everyone should feel attractive and sexy and be told so every day."

"I always flirt, sometimes even with men I am not attracted to, if I feel they need it. I also flirt with women."

ARE YOU JEALOUS?

It is part of his personality to be controlling and that might be perceived as possessive, but most often Cancer is not overtly jealous. There are exceptions to every rule. In all cases, he strives to overcome this negative quality.

"I used to be jealous. I came to understand that I do not own my lovers and I am grateful for any time they choose to spend with me."

"I may be a little jealous, but not much, and I hope my companion is happy enough with me not to go exploring with other guys. I don't monitor his behavior."

"I have been and try not to be."

"Admittedly, very, of everything. I admit that's my problem with my relationships."

HOW DO YOU FEEL ABOUT PUBLIC DISPLAYS OF AFFECTION?

Cancer has a very affectionate nature and when he is in a supportive, accepting place he thinks they are just fine.

"Okay within reason, no frenching in public, holding hands is good."

"I am all for them, but public displays of lust can be tacky . . . get a room."

"It is great, there should be more."

"In a gay-inclusive area, no problem. In the community at large, a kiss, handshake, or hug is okay. I read each situation as it presents itself. I would not want to put my partner or myself at risk."

A MEMORY

"After a superb dinner and great wine we proceeded into a long night of S&M and pain tolerance (me submissive, partner dominant). He worked me over very slowly using restraints—verbal abuse—toys—tit torture—followed by successive golden showers, until I was literally begging him to fuck me into oblivion. Five hours later we both reached orgasm together, after a few others were achieved separately at different heightened awareness."

Sexual Attitudes and Behaviors

HOW OFTEN DO YOU THINK ABOUT SEX AND HOW OFTEN PER WEEK DO YOU WANT TO HAVE SEX?

If there were time, Cancer would have sex daily, perhaps several times per week. Since there isn't that much time, he would like to have sex at least every other day.

"I think about it many times in a day, often dreaming of romantic and wild escapades."

"Having sex every day would be good."

"I would enjoy sex Monday through Friday, morning and night. Weekends: morning, afternoon, and night."

"Sex, as often as reality permits, still have to function in society, go to work, etc."

HOW LONG DO YOU LIKE TO SPEND HAVING SEX AND HOW MUCH OF THAT TIME IS FOREPLAY? DO YOU ENJOY QUICKIES?

Cancer enjoys quick sexual encounters as well as marathon sessions, generally with foreplay lasting about thirty minutes.

"I have spent entire weekends in bed. I also enjoy quickies and everything in between."

"As long as it takes, five minutes to two hours plus."

"Long, short, in between, love, love, love it."

"I enjoy whatever time permits, hours, all night, quickies. How much foreplay depends on the person, his body, and how much time I have."

WHAT TIME OF DAY DO YOU PREFER TO HAVE SEX?

For quickies, any time of day suits him fine. For longer encounters, a bit earlier in the day is preferable to late night.

"Whenever nature takes its course. Mornings are fun. What a great way to start the day, with a smile and pep in my step."

"I enjoy it at any time, whenever I have the opportunity."

HOW OFTEN PER WEEK DO YOU MASTURBATE?

He masturbates on average three times a week.

"I used to love to masturbate while driving fast. I would adjust the rearview mirror so that I could watch myself."

HOW LONG DO YOU WANT TO KNOW SOMEONE BEFORE GETTING SEXUAL?

For Cancer, sex is a natural extension of feeling safe with and close to a man. That may take a few hours or several dates.

"Twenty minutes in a bar—two hours at dinner."

"It used to be a while, like a month or longer, now, 24 hours is sufficient. It depends on how much conversation is involved."

"Depending on how I feel, it could be the same day or two months later."

"Two or three dates, maybe a month."

A MEMORY

"I went to visit my boyfriend, who was in Paris. We had not seen each other for six months. It was 5 a.m., a hot morning. I remember the smells of summer, our hearts pounding, sweaty bodies moving in unison. His musk and the sight of him after so much time kept me completely aroused. We went at it until 2 o'clock in the afternoon and both of us came four times."

WHAT'S YOUR ATTITUDE TOWARD CASUAL SEX?

His only reservations concern practicing safe sex.

"It is my favorite way to make new friends."

"Casual sex is great. It's a real turn on but I use a condom."

"I think it's great but I am in a monogamous relationship so it is not an option now."

DO YOU BELIEVE IN MONOGAMY?

He is capable of being faithful when his sexual needs are met. If sex isn't fulfilling enough with his partner, he is likely to seek it outside.

"I have found love and my life partner. No sharing or other parties are ever required."

"Yes. In a committed relationship, with honesty and trust."

"Yes, commitment develops from mutual trust and respect."

DOES SEX HAVE A SPIRITUAL SIGNIFICANCE FOR YOU?

Cancer is the Sign of home and family. Being in a committed relationship is very rewarding for him, and with such a partner, sex can rise above simple release of sexual tension.

"If it is the right person at the right time and I love that person, then sex is spiritual."

"I seek balance of body, mind, and spirit. Sex plays a role in all three."

"If you love the person, then yes . . . two becoming joined as one being."

"I feel that sex is a very intimate connection, two people sharing of themselves."

FANTASIES

"My partner gets aggressive. I push him away. He forces me to do things to him, it's a little rough, then turns sensual."

"Being worked over by six top leather-clad men, each a master of his own particular area of interest and I being whipped into shape to serve those needs."

ARE YOU COMFORTABLE INITIATING SEXUAL ACTIVITIES?

He has a very strong sex drive and is willing to initiate. A little sexual banter, a slight indication that he won't be rejected flatly, and it's "Your place or mine?"

HOW DO YOU COMMUNICATE TO YOUR PARTNER YOUR SEXUAL WANTS AND NEEDS?

There never needs to be any awkwardness on this subject with Cancer. Sex is so important for this man that he talks about it with ease and wants to be told what his partner most enjoys.

"I usually take what I want, ravage him, and make him feel fabulous."

"We will tell each other what we like and don't like."

"I prefer direct communication, subtle touch, and exploration."

DO YOU THINK OF YOURSELF AS BEING IN THE MAINSTREAM SEXUALLY, MORE EXPERIMENTAL, OR OPEN TO ANYTHING?

Cancer is a very open lover, willing to experiment with bondage, dominance, and submission, sex in public places, water sports, being shaved, and using food along with sex. He prefers sweet tastes such as chocolate. His collection of sex toys may include body clips, butt plugs, dildos, and various restraints.

"I consider myself a sexual outlaw, revolutionary, and pioneer."

"I used to be quite conservative sexually. Now I am open to almost anything. Getting it is a different story."

His fantasies incorporate macho or authoritative men who dominate him.

HOW DO YOU DEMONSTRATE AFFECTION FOR YOUR PARTNER?

He is a romantic. He will leave love notes, buy flowers, cook dinner, or give his lover a massage. He will help around the house and willingly participate in his partner's varied activities.

"I buy him an unexpected treat such as some candy or beverage. I try to make him feel special. I tell him honestly all the things I love about him."

"I do something for him that I know he likes, without his asking, like cleaning the apartment, renting a movie he likes, giving him a massage."

"Write notes, buy flowers, remember special occasions and spontaneous demonstrations of affection."

FANTASIES

"I think of being tied down and restrained forcefully and caressed with a sharp object. In another of my fantasies two men tie me down with chains, then they have their way with me."

"I have always wanted to be tied to the bed and just used."

"For my partner to fuck me silly."

"Being a participant in group sex scenes or a porn video, revisiting past experiences, being a love slave and gang raped."

"A beautiful man sees me across the room and comes over and takes total control."

A MEMORY

"He was quite a bit older and this was our first sexual encounter. He met me at a park and we went for a ride in his car. We stopped in a wooded area and got in the back seat. He was sweaty and smelled like leather. He started touching my groin and pulled it out, stroked a couple of times, and went down. He got up and pulled me toward him and told me to close my eyes. I did. Then he pulled my head down and shoved his dick in my mouth, grabbed my ears, and went to town, moving my head up and down. It took five minutes before he shot his load down my throat and I shot all over him."

The Five Senses

HOW IMPORTANT TO YOU IS THE SEXUAL ENVIRONMENT?

He has a romantic disposition and appreciates a setting designed for sex that is fairly clean, softly lit, and comfortable. Overall, Cancer prefers a place where he will not be interrupted, as he wants to devote his complete attention to the moment and to his partner.

"It's important. On a scale of one to five, it is a four."

"Ambiance is essential. Set the scene to tell your story, whether in the honeymoon suite at the Ritz or behind a Dumpster or on a beach or on the space shuttle."

"Very, but if I am turned on I would do it anywhere."

"A nice place is fine but as long as we are safe from arrest, nothing else matters."

"I never seem to get it as far as lighting and décor, but cleanliness is very important."

WHERE DO YOU LIKE TO HAVE SEX?

Cancer loves his home and the comfort of his bed but variety pleases him. It's a turn-on to get away to a motel or spread a blanket in the woods. Water also often figures in as part of a sexy setting.

"Wherever nature takes it course."

"Outdoors is a turn-on, but my room is best."

"Bedroom and living room so far. I would love to try outdoors."

WHAT PUTS YOU IN THE MOOD FOR SEX?

Cancer is almost always in the mood for sex. Little external stimulation is needed for him to feel ready. Watching videos, such as a good love story, talking about sexual activity, and even talking about past lovers will do the trick as long as those lovers are securely in the past. He is possessive after all.

"Videos, an erotic movie. I am pretty much always in the mood."

"Talking about sexual activity, watching porn videos, fantasizing about a co-worker all put me in the mood."

"A hot man, the sun, summer, erotic movies, baths, and certain smells."

"I am always in the mood for sex. Being outdoors gets me horny, and I like hearing people tell true stories from their sexual past."

"Romantic shows, love music, colognes, watching people dance, coy conversation, provocative apparel."

WHAT'S YOUR ATTITUDE TOWARD PORNOGRAPHY?

He likes pornography, but his taste is very specific. He might enjoy videos that are loving or only those that go beyond vanilla sex or delve into fetishes.

"I love the idea of capturing two beautiful people having great sex and preserving their physical sexual beauty on film as a lasting document, artistic statement, and teaching tool. I don't watch much of it because my reality is hotter than anything I see in porn."

"Love it if it is BDSM, raunchy, bareback, etc. Mainstream is boring."

"I love it. What would we single, action-less people do without it?"

HOW MUCH CUDDLING DO YOU ENJOY, ASIDE FROM SEX?

A hug, an arm around the shoulders, sitting close together while watching TV, and a hand on his knee while driving the car all please Cancer.

A MEMORY

"I met a gorgeous guy in a hot tub. We flirted coyly with each other. I couldn't believe he was into me. When I got out of the tub he followed me to my room and we chatted for a while. The room was warm and dimly lit. I smelled like chlorine so I went to take a shower. After a few minutes he came into the bathroom. We washed each other with scented liquid soap and loofahs. I shampooed his hair then dried him off, touching every inch of him. He teased me by pulling back on a kiss. I grabbed him and pulled him forward. We moved to the bedroom. We kissed and caressed all over. I lay down and he massaged me. Later, after we climaxed, we showered together again."

"I am a cuddly little monkey who likes to touch and be touched."

"Every day . . . twice a day . . . I have to have affection."

HOW TACTILE AND HOW ORAL ARE YOU?

Cancer is all about sensuality, about food, about eating so he is a very oral lover. He also expresses his sensual nature by exploring all parts of his lover's body with his hands.

"The entire human body is a sexual organ, every place on the body has a nerve ending. Touch it, bite it, lick it, pinch it, slap it, poke it, kiss it, rub it, make it feel."

"Very oral. I want to devour my partner with all my senses, taste, smell, see, touch, hear—all bodily fluids are the primordial ooze of the universe and the body has two mouths (mouth and anus); kiss them both."

"Deep kissing on the mouth, lover's body, fellatio."

"Love kissing, rimming is cool. I like using my tongue."

A MEMORY

"I met a beautiful guy out dancing and went back to his place. In addition to being gorgeous he was also sincere and loving. I remember enjoying the smell of his cologne. I gave him a blow job, then we made it into the bedroom. He stretched out on the bed, his beautiful pecs and body before me, as we made love. He was gentle, soft, and kind. It was quite romantic."

WHAT SEX ACTS DO YOU LIKE MOST AND LEAST?

Cancer is open to a wide range of sexual practices, enjoying virtually everything from kissing and oral sex to bondage and dominance and submission role-playing. Rimming is not part of casual sex for him, though he may be willing to try it in a long-term relationship.

"I like kissing, oral sex, intercourse, spanking, and bondage."

"In order: oral sex, anal sex, kissing, and masturbation."

"I love sucking and fucking, deep penetration, opening up and engulfing each other as completely as possible on top and bottom."

AS A LOVER, WHAT'S YOUR BEST SKILL?

Cancer is a nurturing Sign. It is his sensitivity to his partner, rather than any specific sex act, that makes him a particularly skillful lover.

"With me it is my lips and my penis. I always get complimented about those parts of my body."

"Playing their bodies like a musical instrument. After twelve years of active sexuality, I am a virtuoso at playing the human body."

"Deep kissing, and deep-throating a big cock."

"My best skill is my gentle touch with my hands and tongue."

WHAT SMELLS AND TASTES ON YOUR PARTNER DO YOU ENJOY?

He relishes the familiar smells of his lover's body as well as the tastes of his partner's genitals.

"I love the natural smell of his body, it is always the same smell."

"Natural musky smells and tastes, his crotch, pits, breath, sweat, and cum."

"I like the smell and taste of sweat anywhere on his body and I like mixing chocolate into sex play."

"I enjoy the smell of a man's skin and cologne, his shampoo and soap, the taste of freshly showered skin, and a man's tongue if he is not a smoker."

FOR SOME PEOPLE THE TASTE OF THEIR PARTNER'S CUM IS UNPLEASANT. IF THAT'S TRUE FOR YOU, WHAT DO YOU DO ABOUT THE TASTE?

In a casual relationship he is unlikely to ingest cum, more for health reasons than having to do with taste. In a long-term relationship if he finds the taste objectionable, he will strive to avoid having his partner climax in his mouth.

"I try not to taste it because I am concerned about STDs."

"I don't mind precum, but I don't like the taste of cum. I prefer my partner to cum on my face and chest and I use it as a lube to jerk off."

MEMORIES

"Partner blindfolds me and ties me up, pulling me, fisting me, and I cum without ever touching myself."

"I love dancing with my partner, smelling his skin, dancing for hours, running him home, cuddling, slow sex, then sleeping."

"Driving in the country, past a good-looking guy. I pulled over. It was so intense. He smelled of great cologne. My other favorite memories are being outside in nature and having wild, passionate sex."

"I don't taste my partner's for safety reasons. I do taste my own and I like it."

"I don't like the taste at all. I use mouthwash before going down."

DO YOU ENJOY WATCHING YOUR PARTNER DURING SEX AND ORGASM? DO YOU ENJOY BEING WATCHED?

He is thoroughly comfortable with intimacy. Eye contact intensifies the sense of connection that he feels during sex. He is totally at ease both watching and being watched by his partner.

"Absolutely. I am both an exhibitionist and a voyeur."

"I feel awkward at first being watched, but over time I come to enjoy it."

The Big "O"
• •

HOW DO YOU REACH AN ORGASM AND HOW OFTEN?

He achieves orgasm with ease through such sex acts as oral and anal sex and masturbation.

"Orally and masturbation. I enjoy orgasm the best while my lover is fucking me."

"It could be anything, even mutual masturbation."

"I achieve orgasm most of the time, but I am not 'goal oriented.' I am more interested in getting my partner off and I love to cum and then keep going."

WHAT'S YOUR FAVORITE POSITION?

His favorite positions include doggie style and 69.

"On my back, kissing a man with my finger up my ass, his weight on top of me, me jacking off, while he squeezes my balls, or any position with a huge cock down my throat."

SOME PEOPLE ARE CONCERNED ABOUT BRINGING A PARTNER TO CLIMAX BEFORE HAVING AN ORGASM THEMSELVES. OTHERS STRIVE TO REACH ORGASM TOGETHER. WHICH IS TRUE FOR YOU?

Cancer's only concern is that both he and his lover are ultimately satisfied. Who comes first is not significant.

"As long as we both have our orgasm I will be happy. I will make sure we do."

"Who cums first is not a problem for my partner or me. It is about the journey not the destination."

"Each of us climaxes whenever we are ready."

ARE YOU VOCAL DURING SEX?

He is highly vocal during sex, communicating both his appreciation for his lover and the level of his excitement.

"How vocal I am during sex depends on the scene, usually lots of moans and slurps. I get very chatty and philosophical during sex, so sometimes you have to put something in my mouth to shut me up."

AFTER SEX WHAT DO YOU LIKE TO DO?

After sex he'll want something to eat. What that is depends upon the time of day. It might be a snack in the kitchen or dinner out, but either way, food is the best way to finish off the experience.

"I hold my partner and kiss him and tell him I enjoyed his company."

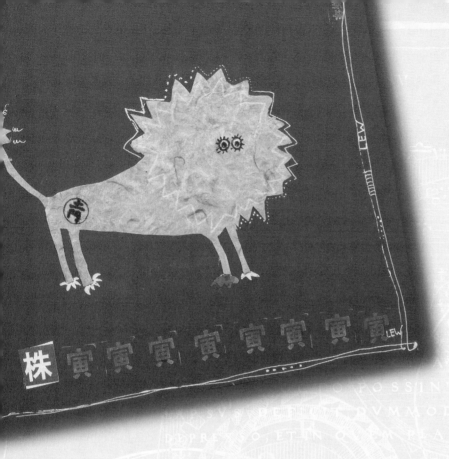

Leo
THE LION

July 23 through August 22

FIRE SIGN LEO has a sunny, generous disposition, is flamboyant, enthusiastic, and loves having an audience. Ruler of the spine and heart, Leo is a romantic for whom setting the stage for sex is important. Cleanliness, a candle or two, and some flowers enhance the Lion's sexual pleasure.

What he says: "I lightly run my fingers down his back to his ass, and rub it lightly and using my tongue from chest, nipples to penis to drive him into a complete moaning frenzy."

"I never miss a chance to have sex or appear on television."

—Gore Vidal

The Leo Man
in His Own Words

"We were lying naked on the sand dunes in Provincetown, Massachusetts. warmed by the afternoon sun. The only sound was the rhythmic crashing of waves and my lover's breath in my ear. I remember the feeling of my lover's body wrapped around me like a serpent. We kissed for long periods, barely able to breathe from passion. I just wanted to eat him whole. We became one body of sensation slathered in sweat made more slippery by precum. The level was so intense, building for hours, to the point that neither of us needed to even touch each other's penis to achieve orgasm. It happened just through rubbing against each other while kissing."

Attraction and Dating a Leo

WHAT ATTRACTS YOU TO SOMEONE?

For Leo, "all the world's a stage," so to catch Leo's attention first of all, a handsome face and a fit physique is a must. In fact, he takes something of a physical inventory head to toe, and when he has the chance to have sex with a new partner, penis size does matter to him.

"Eyes first! Then his mouth, stomach, hands, neck, plus intelligence, compassion, mannerisms, and ability to communicate."

"Maturity, honesty, ones personality, physique. A man's looks are somewhat of a factor, hair and penis."

"Body, eyes, hair, energy, masculinity, butt."

"Masculinity, large penis size, facial hair, self-confidence, short hair."

"Muscles, eyes, nice buttocks, sexy body language, flirtatious behavior, eye contact, smile, friendly."

"I love muscular men with pretty faces who are cheerful, outgoing, and confident."

"A man's brain, his muscles, smell, manly attitude, good looks."

WHAT MIGHT TURN YOU OFF?

Leo is a man who likes being the center of attention; therefore, a person who focuses primarily upon himself will always turn him off. In addition, when one is in the limelight, being well groomed is important, so the man who goes out in grubby sweats or overly casual jeans won't hold Leo's attention for very long.

"I am put off by conceited egomaniacs and definitely poor grooming."

"Number one turn-off, not being real, a liar, overweight, smoking, drinking."

"Some behaviors, like being overly effeminate."

"Overbearing, needs to have the center of attention about him all the time."

"Snobbishness, being unfit, sloppy dresser, bad teeth, odor."

"Selfish or snobby personalities, cocky people, and people who smell. It is sad how many people have poor hygiene."

WHAT DO YOU ENJOY DOING ON A DATE?

Leo is a high energy Sign. On a date he prefers to be out in public in a group. He loves conversing with many people. He'll enjoy active dates—miniature golfing, ocean walks, hiking, biking, or going to amusement parks. He also likes the traditional dinner or a film.

"Conversation is most enjoyable, getting to know a man to see if there is a connection."

"Movies, talk about significant and insignificant things without feeling awkward."

"Going to a nice restaurant, chatting, a nice Pinot, then go out for a beer, and dance."

"Movie, music, dancing, dining, drinking, conversation."

"Nice dinner, a play rather than a movie, visit a museum, or go to a music festival."

"Getting to know the individual, perhaps over dinner, talking in a quiet place, either at home or in the car."

"Talking, I love to get to know the other person over a meal, a walk, or even sitting on a barstool having a drink."

ARE YOU FLIRTATIOUS?

He is outgoing, extremely friendly, and quite flirtatious. In fact Leo has an ability to enter a room and take center stage quite effortlessly. He loves the attention he gets from others. After all, Leo is the Lion and relishes having his mane stroked.

"Flirtatious? Extremely!"

"Oh yes. I flirt every chance I get."

"Yes. Well, it depends on who is judging, I think I am somewhat flirtatious. Some people think I flirt a lot."

ARE YOU JEALOUS?

Ever the performer, naturally in control, easily taking center stage, Leo can be jealous simply because he expects to be fully attended to by his partner.

"I get jealous sometimes, especially when my partner's old boyfriend is pulling strings."

"Oh yes. If I see someone I want and someone else wants him too."

"Yes, too much for my own good."

"I am, at first, when I am developing a relationship, but that passes once I am confident my partner and I are into one another."

A FANTASY

"I get pulled over by a strikingly handsome state trooper who forces me to have sex with him in order to avoid getting a ticket. In my mind the situation must trigger an element of fear, a sensation that I have little or no control. This leads to him contacting me in the future for more of the same."

HOW DO YOU FEEL ABOUT PUBLIC DISPLAYS OF AFFECTION?

Leo is a performer. To some extent he is always on stage and expects to get attention from the audience. He enjoys observing and participating in moderate displays of affection, as long as the environment is safe and gay friendly.

"Public displays of affection are good for everybody, the recipients, as well as onlookers. We display violence so easily, yet forcefully oppress affection. Why?"

"Holding hands is great, kissing is okay, but swallowing face is not acceptable."

"In clubs it's all right, other than that I don't participate."

"They are okay if done in small ways. I am not fond of excessive public displays of affection."

"Yes, when it is appropriate."

"Proper displays at proper times are nice."

Sexual Attitudes and Behaviors

A MEMORY

"One of the best sexual encounters I ever had was with my long-term partner after a night out. The sex was rough and felt better than any I'd had in a very long time. And yet, it was also romantic, because of the love we felt for one another."

HOW OFTEN DO YOU THINK ABOUT SEX AND HOW OFTEN PER WEEK DO YOU WANT TO HAVE SEX?

It fits with his flirtatious nature that he sees sexual innuendoes in many different activities, so he thinks about sex frequently in the course of a day. He wants to have sex four times a week.

"I think about sex several times daily. I guess I am pre-occupied with it. Aren't most men?"

"As a general rule, I want sex all the time. Okay, I must admit, sometimes I would rather sleep."

HOW LONG DO YOU LIKE TO SPEND HAVING SEX AND HOW MUCH OF THAT TIME IS FOREPLAY? DO YOU ENJOY QUICKIES?

He enjoys spending about three-quarters of an hour having sex, as well as the occasional quickie. As to foreplay, he likes spending twenty to thirty minutes.

"I prefer at least an hour, but I do find 'hit and runs' erotic."

"Quickies are great, but long sessions are the best."

"I like to have forty minutes. Quickies . . . it depends. If we are in a hurry, then they are okay."

"Taking our time is the best. Ultimately that makes for a much more intense build up and a more satisfying orgasm follows."

"Sometimes playing around can be the entire event."

WHAT TIME OF DAY DO YOU PREFER TO HAVE SEX?

While he isn't likely to say "no" in the morning or at night, his preference is for late afternoon or early evening.

"What time of day don't I want sex?"

"I love afternoon, with no time constraints."

"I really enjoy late afternoon, otherwise just about any-time is fine."

A FANTASY

"I love the image of having sex with a smooth muscle boy in a locker room. He is all sweaty, wearing just a jock strap or spandex briefs. I lick the sweat out of his butt and savor smelling it. I love the smell of sweat. I rim him and lick his body, then have intercourse, and rub our bodies together, smelling his jock or spandex, kissing or making love."

HOW OFTEN PER WEEK DO YOU MASTURBATE?

He masturbates four or five times a week.

HOW LONG DO YOU WANT TO KNOW SOMEONE BEFORE GETTING SEXUAL?

Leo is a Sign that acts on instinct and he trusts this feeling in his response to a new man. In most circumstances, as soon as he realizes that the other is available or open to the suggestion, he is ready to become sexual. Usually this occurs on the first or at the latest on the second date. On occasion he may wait a few more dates.

"No amount of time is required, maybe about five minutes. It just really depends on the guy and the situation."

"It can be right away. But when I start talking with a man and realize there's a strong connection and the possibility of a serious relationship, I wait through several dates."

"Shorter rather than longer, usually."

WHAT'S YOUR ATTITUDE TOWARD CASUAL SEX?

Is it risky? Sure. Does he care? Yes, enough to take precautions but then he'll go for it.

"I think anonymous sex is fine, but in fact sex is better when you care about your partner."

A MEMORY

"My partner invited a friend for a weekend of sex and he included me in on it. We went to dinner and had some drinks in very stylish and sexy locales. I was extremely aggressive, kissing both of them at dinner in public, and dirty dancing with this friend. Later back home, I went to town on him, no problem with my partner. I had really hot sex with both of them and we did it again in the morning."

DO YOU BELIEVE IN MONOGAMY?

Flirt that he is and charmer that he is, many opportunities present themselves, and he acknowledges that having sex with the same man all the time is not easy to maintain. Nevertheless, he wants to be in a monogamous relationship.

"Being in a long-term relationship, you can grow with another person and you do not feel the need to impress anyone except the one you love."

"Yes, in a sense. However, if there is consent between the partners to involve others sexually, that can still work within the relationship."

"I believe that everyone is capable of monogamy, but some people have overactive sex drives and find it difficult to resist temptations."

"Yes, eventually two people should only want to be with each other, to just see each other in a sexual, loving way."

"I feel better in a committed relationship. Knowing my partner is only with me feels so safe."

"Yes, when a couple wants to commit to each other it is a beautiful thing."

DOES SEX HAVE A SPIRITUAL SIGNIFICANCE FOR YOU?

Without a doubt. For Leo, with all his exuberance and desire to be adored, which can lead to lots of casual sex, what gives him the greatest sexual pleasure is the kind of passion only felt in a committed relationship. He sees this as spiritual.

"God gave us this wonderful gift, to please one another. Sex with someone you're committed to is a higher high than I had ever anticipated."

"Sex is a bonding between two individuals. There is nothing else like it."

"Real intimacy is spiritual."

"Yes, my soul feels bonded to the other person."

ARE YOU COMFORTABLE INITIATING SEXUAL ACTIVITIES?

Leo is naturally outgoing and confident. He seldom has any trouble initiating a physical relationship. On the contrary, with his charm and openness he can broach this subject in such a way that a refusal won't feel like a rejection.

HOW DO YOU COMMUNICATE TO YOUR PARTNER YOUR SEXUAL WANTS AND NEEDS?

Leo is a Fire Sign, known for his ability to move with cat-like grace. When it comes to talking about sex, he prefers to let his body do the work. Though he may use some words to direct his partner, he is more likely to communicate with gestures or by moving his lover's hand.

"More often than using words, I communicate through kisses and by rubbing my body against my lover."

"I use mostly gestures and moans. I only use words on occasion."

"Both, though I wish I were better at the words."

"When we get into bed, I start to rub his body. Sometimes I ask him to make love to me."

DO YOU THINK OF YOURSELF AS BEING IN THE MAINSTREAM SEXUALLY, MORE EXPERIMENTAL, OR OPEN TO ANYTHING?

This is a man who loves to play, to perform. When it comes to sex, he is an experimental lover open to sex in public places, ménage à trois, exhibitionism, dominance and submission, voyeurism, using costumes, and spanking. In addition, a lover who introduces another element with a sense of fun will find a willing partner in Leo.

In his fantasies the normally dominant Leo usually plays a submissive role in a scene that involves multiple partners.

A FANTASY

"Having sex with two people, one oral, the other doggie style, getting fucked. I love to handle two big dicks at once. My fantasy is like my favorite porn movie, 'The Biggest I Ever Saw,' a '70s film. All of the guys were at least 9 inches."

HOW DO YOU DEMONSTRATE AFFECTION FOR YOUR PARTNER?

He is a thoughtful lover who strives to show appreciation with cards, notes, flowers, and perhaps by cooking dinners. He is a romantic in so many ways, but doesn't necessarily attend to the calendar to observe that it is an anniversary or even a birthday, but they are important to him. A caring lover will bring up the subject of approaching important dates.

"With thoughtfulness, I include them in my life process and decision making where appropriate."

"Bringing small gifts, saying 'I love you' kissing, cuddling, complimenting, using pet names."

"I am always polite, caring, and compassionate towards his feelings. I love to touch and fondle him."

"I may cook a fancy meal, strew rose petals from the doorway of the house to the foot of the bed, massage his tender feet when he is tired."

The Five Senses

HOW IMPORTANT TO YOU IS THE SEXUAL ENVIRONMENT?

Comfort counts so a soft bed, even if the sheets haven't been changed terribly recently, is important to him. It isn't that cleanliness is completely irrelevant, but as a general rule, the setting for sex is not of great consequence to Leo and experimenting in unusual settings can add fun.

"Somewhat important, I prefer comfort."

"I have had sex in everything . . . in underground sewers and in chapels, so apparently the environment is not very important to me."

"It is not crucial, but anything that enhances the experience is a bonus."

"If you get me at the right time, it is not important at all."

WHERE DO YOU LIKE TO HAVE SEX?

Any place private. Leo may flirt and be something of an exhibitionist but most often with his clothes on. In other words he doesn't want to be observed by strangers when having sex. If he is going to have sex in a somewhat public place, it needs to be in a secluded area.

"I like having sex in our bedroom but also enjoy the fun of sex in unexpected locations with the exception of places where it could be dangerous and we might get arrested. Otherwise, I am up for sex just about anywhere."

"Warm dunes on the beach."

"Hotel rooms, sex clubs, and public, meaning outdoor spaces, discreet of course."

"Anywhere, even outside, but not so public that we might be seen."

"I prefer being inside a house, no particular room. Other places are not out of the question, they just aren't as comfortable."

FANTASIES

"They all consist of a large, muscular man, taking complete control of me, not in an S&M kind of way, just dominating me until we both orgasm."

"I imagine a three or four way scene including my partner in our bed or on the floor. That's all it takes, just the image of us four naked men."

A MEMORY

"We were on a dark bus, late at night, and only the two of us were sitting on the back seat. I had dozed off. My partner took me in his arms and started to kiss me awake. He opened my zipper and began to blow me. There were only the sounds of the engine, the smell of his body odor, and of our love."

WHAT PUTS YOU IN THE MOOD FOR SEX?

A little flirting, a little exhibitionism, then get his senses going with good food, conversation, or music and he's in the mood.

"When the wind blows with the light lavender scent in the air . . . in other words, it doesn't take too much."

"Stimulating conversation over a luscious meal, followed by any tactile activity, such as caressing and kissing."

"Romantic sexy music, close contact, natural male aroma, champagne or good wine, tender and then heated touching and rubbing, sexy clothing and underwear."

"Incense, porn, showering, massage, dirty talk whispered in my ear."

"Music, I prefer techno, some aromas, such as the smell of his skin, pornography too, a touch."

"Just being close to my partner and cuddling is enough, but visual stimuli, whether it be him or TV or movies will work too."

WHAT'S YOUR ATTITUDE TOWARD PORNOGRAPHY?

Without exception every Leo loves pornography. He enjoys it in many forms, from erotic literature to sleazy magazines and a full range of videos from mild to wild.

HOW MUCH CUDDLING DO YOU ENJOY ASIDE FROM SEX?

There is no doubt that Leo enjoys a considerable amount of cuddling aside from sex, but there is a fine line between cuddling and clinging. Clinging is possessive and no Lion will be possessed.

"A lot. I can fall asleep in someone's arms with the right kind of cuddling."

"Sometimes just holding and caressing is fantastic."

"I love cuddling, it is very romantic to be held."

"I love to snuggle and cuddle."

"I like lots of cuddling. I love romantic touch and contact."

HOW TACTILE AND HOW ORAL ARE YOU?

Leo has a take charge personality and likes to prove his prowess in bed by turning his partner on with his tactile skills. Using both mouth and hands, he touches every part of his lover's skin.

"I am extremely tactile, I just don't stop."

"A lot, absolutely, I am very touchy, feely, romantic."

"I cover every square inch with my mouth."

"Very oral, kissing, fellatio, love rimming and devouring my partner's body with kisses."

WHAT SEX ACTS DO YOU LIKE MOST AND LEAST?

He has a flamboyant nature and is quite experimental in his willingness to explore sexual behaviors. Leo's favorite sex acts include oral sex, kissing, and masturbation and beyond that, mixing in a costume, or participating in a threesome heightens the playful aspect of sex. When it comes to anal sex generally he likes either giving or receiving, not both.

"I like giving anal sex though I do not like receiving it."

"I like masturbation, giving oral, getting rimmed, and fucked."

"I do not like anal intercourse where I penetrate."

AS A LOVER, WHAT'S YOUR BEST SKILL?

Most of all, what makes Leo a good lover is his desire to take charge and thoroughly please his lover.

"I lightly run my fingers down his back, to his ass and rub it lightly and using my tongue from chest, nipples to penis to drive him into a complete moaning frenzy."

"Blow jobs, great tongue, mouth, deep throat action."

> **A FANTASY**
>
> "In the dungeon, as I inspect the prisoners, I notice this little blonde bottom boy in a harness. I pick him out to be put on the stretcher, not to torture him physically, but sexually. He starts screaming that I will kill him, but I put my mouth on his member as he calms down. I play with his nipples as he cums down my throat. Then I proceed to bathe him tenderly, all the while sticking my finger up his ass to loosen him up. He wiggles with anticipation."

"Would have to say tongue. I give great fellatio."

"Use of my tongue and beard."

"Touch, very sensual feel, great kisser, and use of tongue."

WHAT SMELLS AND TASTES ON YOUR PARTNER DO YOU ENJOY?

Leo loves his partner's clean and also sweaty aroma, as well as the masculine smells of armpits and crotch. He also likes the taste of his partner's lips, skin, and sex organs.

"Clean slightly sweaty smells with a trace of colognes."

"I love his body odor."

"Love masculine smells and tastes, armpits, anus, crotch, and chest."

"Male body odor, some sweat, light clean soapy smell, or minty cologne."

"I love the sweat on his back as it trickles down after sex."

A MEMORY

"After ending a six-year relationship, I was feeling depressed and decided to return to a favorite cruising spot at a local movie theater that I used to frequent before my relationship. I met an acquaintance from my past. We talked for a while, then proceeded to a video booth, where we attacked each other aggressively. The flicker of a gay porn movie was the only light. The aroma of sex and poppers filled my nostrils. The heat, the confinement of the booth, the darkness, and the animalistic lust has made this experience the most memorable and extraordinary for me."

FOR SOME PEOPLE THE TASTE OF THEIR PARTNER'S CUM IS UNPLEASANT. IF THAT'S TRUE FOR YOU, HOW DO YOU HANDLE IT?

He doesn't like the taste of cum and wants his partner to avoid cumming in his mouth.

"I never swallow, don't like the taste. Shoot it anywhere but down my throat."

"Swallow some, rub some on my cock to masturbate with."

"I never swallow but occasionally rub it on myself."

DO YOU ENJOY WATCHING YOUR PARTNER DURING SEX AND ORGASM? DO YOU ENJOY BEING WATCHED?

He loves to watch his partner during sex and orgasm and is equally comfortable being watched. In addition, the performer in Leo is not above observing his own performance in a well-placed mirror.

The Big "O"

HOW DO YOU REACH AN ORGASM AND HOW OFTEN?

Leo usually reaches orgasm through masturbation, sometimes with oral or anal sex.

"Through oral sex and masturbation, I cum all the time, at least two times."

"I almost always reach orgasm and by my own hand. I derive pleasure out of satisfying another, while masturbating, or deep kissing, and mutual masturbation."

"Hopefully while he is fucking me."

WHAT'S YOUR FAVORITE POSITION?

There are many that he enjoys but most often his preference is doggie style.

"Fucking from behind and deep kissing and masturbation face to face."

"I like sitting on his dick while he lies down."

FANTASIES

"My sex fantasies always involve group sex with me as the bottom, being tag-team fucked, the center of attention, pleasing multiple partners."

"Usually if I see a guy I like, I fantasize about him wearing some kind of uniform, such as UPS deliveryman, policeman, or construction worker."

"Images include rimming. I love the anus and a great butt. I'm with guys who have well-developed arm and leg muscles and who at times manhandle me. At other times I am the dominant one."

SOME PEOPLE ARE CONCERNED ABOUT BRINGING A PARTNER TO CLIMAX BEFORE HAVING AN ORGASM THEMSELVES. OTHERS STRIVE TO REACH ORGASM TOGETHER. WHICH IS TRUE FOR YOU?

For Leo the idea of mutual orgasm is more of a hope than an objective. He is the King of the Jungle and like any good monarch he is generous to his subjects. He wants to please his partner.

"I always make sure he climaxes. I want him to be fulfilled."

"It varies, but usually my partner first."

"Bring partner to orgasm first, then I masturbate."

"Hopefully mutual, otherwise partner first."

"I strive to reach orgasm together."

"I like us to reach it at the same time."

ARE YOU VOCAL DURING SEX?

Most often he is only slightly vocal although there are some Leo men who really let it all out.

"All I say is 'Fuck me, Fuck me.'"

"We scare people."

AFTER SEX WHAT DO YOU LIKE TO DO?

Sex sometimes energizes him and he wants to go out, especially if it is fairly early in the day or evening. Most of the time, however, he prefers to relax and stay home. Either way, he wants to take his time between sex and other activities. This is when, most of all, he likes to cuddle for a bit.

"Kiss, cuddle, talk, fall asleep in each others arms."

"Sleep, relax, eat, nap together, and watch TV."

"Cuddle then go out to a movie and dinner."

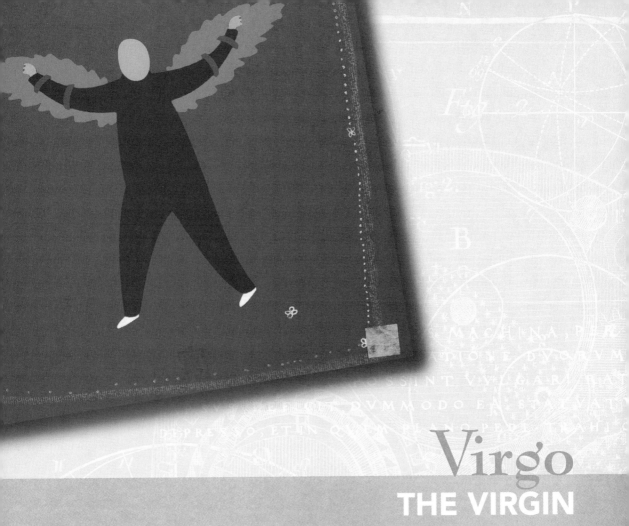

Virgo
THE VIRGIN

August 23 through September 22

"Cleanliness is next to Godliness."

—John Wesley, Sermon 93,
"On Dress"

EARTH SIGN VIRGO is straightforward, a devoted friend, very physical, and works hard at everything he does, including sexually fulfilling a partner. Virgo, ruler of the abdomen and bowels, health and hygiene, is attracted by a man who is in very good physical condition.

What he says: "I am very oral, I think giving head to a guy is one of the sexiest things in the world."

The Virgo Man in His Own Words

A MEMORY

"Having sex in our garage on a hot summer day. We were sweaty and a little dirty. We opened a sling-back lawn chair and he straddled me. He stuck his big fat dick in my mouth. I felt his balls slapping against my chin. The sweat dripped off him and he started to moan as he came in my mouth."

Attraction and Dating a Virgo

WHAT ATTRACTS YOU TO SOMEONE?

Virgo is something of a hypochondriac and has the reputation for being a neat freak. In fact, his house may be sloppy, but someone who is not well groomed or neatly dressed in public will never get his attention. In addition, to attract a Virgo, a man must exude an aura of good physical health.

"Overall health, intelligence, social consciousness, responsibility, humor, creativity, respect for others."

"Well groomed, nice hair, lovely teeth, in shape body."

"Imagination, confidence, and kindness, someone I can trust to respect me."

"Lots of body hair and meaty thighs. I love big cocks but that's not a necessity, and a really nice ass."

WHAT MIGHT TURN YOU OFF?

The physical traits that he dislikes include poor dental hygiene and being overweight. But a bad attitude is the major turn-off for Virgo.

"Insensitivity, crass behavior, being 'full of himself,' and using drugs definitely repel me."

"Arrogance, obesity, cynicism, dependence, and unhealthy behaviors."

"Men who are overly dominant, ignorance."

A MEMORY

"I was on vacation in Florida with a dear friend. It was hot, a light breeze blowing. We went for a swim. No one else was in the pool, though a few people were lounging, no children. We were horsing around and I was horny. He squeezed my nipples, and that drives me crazy. Then he turned around and held on to the side of the pool. I came up behind him and straddled him, my chest pressing against his back, my penis hard, hanging out of the leg of my swim trunks. I moved my hips back and forth, rubbing my dick on the smooth nylon of his Speedos. I am easily stimulated and this was enough to make me cum in just a few minutes."

WHAT DO YOU ENJOY DOING ON A DATE?

Virgo has a quiet disposition and for a date he prefers easygoing activities, such as dinners at home or out with friends. It doesn't matter whether he's with someone new or a long-standing partner.

"Conversation, a long walk, holding hands, enjoying each other's company."

"Movies, dinner, quiet evening maybe just watching TV, maybe sex, but not necessarily on the first date."

"Sharing food, talking, a drive through a park or to the ocean."

"Dancing and quiet activities such as going to an art gallery or a museum."

ARE YOU FLIRTATIOUS?

Given that Virgo is a reserved Sign, his flirtatiousness is subtle at best. He may wish that he was more relaxed, especially in approaching someone he finds attractive.

"I am, but still pretty reserved about it."

"Yes, but very subtly, on a scale of one to ten, a five."

"It depends on my own insecurity, I flirt when I need."

ARE YOU JEALOUS?

Jealousy is not a fundamental trait of this Sign. If a man goes out of his way and succeeds in making him jealous, Virgo will be unhappy with himself and angry at his lover's behavior, resulting in less, not more, attention from Virgo.

"I could be if given enough cause."

"I am sometimes, but working on it."

"I can be. With my current boyfriend, I never felt jealous until I found him expressing suspicion toward me. It made me feel like maybe he was hiding something. So I found myself becoming highly suspicious and jealous of some of his connections with other people."

HOW DO YOU FEEL ABOUT PUBLIC DISPLAYS OF AFFECTION?

Virgo is a Sign that is known to be particular and discreet. As a result, while he likes public displays he uses caution.

"I think they're wonderful. They beat public displays of war and inhumanity that we're inundated with."

"I don't mind, if they're not too overt."

"Love it unless in a threatening environment."

"I prefer to be subtle, but in erotic situations, a club, the baths, I am exhibitionistic."

> ### A FANTASY
>
> "An aggressive police officer stops my car, takes me to an isolated spot, pulls out his very long, thick penis and orders me to perform oral sex. He forcefully thrusts into my mouth and deep into my throat as he cums."

Sexual Attitudes and Behaviors

HOW OFTEN DO YOU THINK ABOUT SEX AND HOW OFTEN PER WEEK DO YOU WANT TO HAVE SEX?

Sex is frequently on his mind if he's not preoccupied with it. He'd like to have sex every day but will be content with three to five times a week.

"I think about sex hourly, it's my favorite thing."

"When I have a steady partner I want sex at least once a day."

HOW LONG DO YOU LIKE TO SPEND HAVING SEX AND HOW MUCH OF THAT TIME IS FOREPLAY? DO YOU ENJOY QUICKIES?

He prefers spending up to an hour for sex, occasionally longer and quickies are fine with him. Foreplay varies widely, from ten to forty-five minutes, depending on his mood.

"I enjoy quickies, but thirty minutes to an hour does it for me."

"An hour at the most, quickies sometimes at the beach."

"Regarding foreplay, no more than ten minutes. If he doesn't want me by then, forget it."

A FANTASY

"I fantasize about interracial sex with two very masculine men dressed as cops. Lots of lovemaking, passion, and kissing, not rough, just experimental. The men would have large penises and I would be receiving them."

WHAT TIME OF DAY DO YOU PREFER TO HAVE SEX?

This is a man who works hard at everything that he does. He wants to please his partner, therefore he wants sex when he isn't overly tired. Evenings are nice before a night out. Mornings can be fine prior to leaving for work.

HOW OFTEN PER WEEK DO YOU MASTURBATE?

He masturbates six times per week.

HOW LONG DO YOU WANT TO KNOW SOMEONE BEFORE GETTING SEXUAL?

Virgo may not be in a major hurry to get sexual, but he doesn't want to wait very long. He wants to feel comfortable, sure that a man is healthy, and that may take a few weeks. There are times when he throws his usual caution aside and leaps into a sexual relationship at once.

"There's too much pressure to have sex on the first date. Maybe the second date."

"That depends on whether he's husband material or just pretty."

"I've had sex on the first date but also waited weeks. Most often, the second or third date works for me."

"I don't need to know a man at all for sex. For a relationship, I want to know him at least three to four months."

WHAT'S YOUR ATTITUDE TOWARD CASUAL SEX?

One might expect health-conscious Virgo to shy away from casual sex. Not so.

"I love it, I think sex is underrated."

"I love it when single, but it's out of the question now that I have a partner."

"It is unsafe, but it happens."

DO YOU BELIEVE IN MONOGAMY?

He does.

"I desire it for myself and I believe it's possible."

"Nothing is more fulfilling than a monogamous long-term relationship. It shows respect for my partner."

"Yes, you won't be distracted. Monogamy provides that 100 percent security."

But a little sex on the side is okay.

"Relationships can be monogamous and still be open sexually."

"I don't think a quickie with someone else should hurt a partnership."

"I believe in it but I've been in an open relationship for twelve years."

FANTASIES

"One of my fantasies is having two men at the same time. No costumes or kink, just all three of us totally naked on a shag rug. I think being on my hands and knees, sucking off a guy, while another one does me doggie style could make me cum without either of them giving my cock even one stroke."

"Love the idea of seducing and turning on a straight guy. Fucking body builders. Having a woman want to have sex with me even though I am gay. Having sex with a stranger from the gym."

"I enjoy the thought of my partner servicing other men. While I find the idea upsetting, it is highly arousing. I'd love to watch my partner sucking off another guy or being fucked by another guy. I would love to sit in the same room and just watch them, even instruct them."

DOES SEX HAVE A SPIRITUAL SIGNIFICANCE FOR YOU?

Given the practical nature of an Earth Sign, casual sex remains purely physical to Virgo. In a serious and deeply loving relationship, however, sex transcends to something more.

"In my current relationship, sex has been spiritual. We are realizing another level of understanding of each other."

"I believe it's one of the highest connections between two human beings, a celebration of our bodies, of joy, and of the life force."

"Yes, if in a monogamous relationship. I feel each sexual act contributes to the spiritual connection that we share."

ARE YOU COMFORTABLE INITIATING SEXUAL ACTIVITIES?

It's not about fear of rejection, more a fundamental part of his nature that he would prefer the other to take charge. He isn't likely to say no but all in all, he doesn't want to initiate the conversation or the act.

"It's not that I am uncomfortable doing it, but I prefer not initiating sex."

"I am not very aggressive."

"Sometimes. I am getting better at it, but I prefer for him to start."

A MEMORY

"A three way with my partner and a tight muscular guy dressed in leather, at his apartment. He lit candles, had porno on. We drank each other's piss, fucked each other, and came a lot, relaxed a bit and then went out to dinner."

HOW DO YOU COMMUNICATE TO YOUR PARTNER YOUR SEXUAL WANTS AND NEEDS?

Earth Sign Virgo is quite straightforward on the topic of sex. He may be a bit subtle with a new partner, but in a very short time, he will let his pleasure be known clearly with both words and gestures.

"I touch him or simply tell him. We are very comfortable that way."

"We speak very openly about sex."

DO YOU THINK OF YOURSELF AS BEING IN THE MAINSTREAM SEXUALLY, MORE EXPERIMENTAL, OR OPEN TO ANYTHING?

He usually stays within a range of sexuality from mainstream to somewhat experimental, performing oral and anal sex, ménage à trois, and using toys such as dildoes, cock rings, vibrators, penis pumps, and butt plugs, and occasionally using uniforms in sex play. Beyond that he may be open to using food, less frequently ice cubes and hot wax, exhibitionism, and group sex.

"I only use sex toys when I am single. I own several dildoes including one that supposedly has a lifelike orgasm button. I even had a 'mannequin man,' a male love doll."

The most open Virgos, few in number, are willing to try bondage, dominance, and submission, and occasionally sadomasochism using such toys as whips, chains, or cock and ball torture.

Virgo's fantasies generally involve oral sex and anal penetration and sometimes group or anonymous sex.

FANTASIES

"I imagine getting fucked by six or eight guys and they all cum in my ass . . . group showers and guys jerking off all over me. Thick fat cock in my mouth with a lot of cum."

"Having sex with a bisexual hairy man in an eighteen-wheeler. He is sitting in the driver's seat and I am facing him, sitting on his cock, and feeling his big hairy chest and deep kissing him all at the same time. And yes, I have a hard-on while I am writing this."

HOW DO YOU DEMONSTRATE AFFECTION FOR YOUR PARTNER?

Virgo may be more pragmatic than he is romantic, giving gifts that are utilitarian rather than touching little tokens, but he is consistently attentive and aware when his partner needs his assistance.

"Lots of touching aside from sex, being sincere, generous, patient, concerned."

"Being supportive, making his favorite meal, listening when he speaks."

"We always say we love each other. I do nice things for him. I am a great listener."

"Making and serving special foods, kind words, and buying things he likes."

MEMORIES

"After a huge fight with a lover we reconciled by spending one full day together in bed. We only left the bed to eat or go to the bathroom. We had sex repeatedly throughout the entire day."

"Performing oral sex on a very well-endowed stranger in a public restroom. The anonymity, being a pure sexual object to him, putting him into ecstasy, making him cum in my mouth, having him in awe of how good I made him feel all add up to this extraordinary encounter."

"It was the first time my boyfriend ever had sex with me. He asked me to wear a blindfold. He let me touch his body , and I found that all he had on was leather-wear, a hat, a vest, chaps, and boots. It was very hot. After a lot of foreplay the sex lasted for hours."

The Five Senses

● ●

HOW IMPORTANT TO YOU IS THE SEXUAL ENVIRONMENT?

Beyond cleanliness, the setting for sex is of little importance to Virgo. With his matter-of-fact nature, Virgo's focus is exclusively on the act and his partner.

"I can have sex anywhere, but a pretty setting makes it more romantic."

"Environment has nothing to do with it for me. I like a clean place, but my partner's positive attitude and concern for me is most important."

"The environment has its place, but I rule nothing out."

"Cleanliness is important, otherwise the environment doesn't matter to me, as long as it is not a total sty."

WHERE DO YOU LIKE TO HAVE SEX?

Safety makes Virgo feel more relaxed, so his favorite place for sex is at home. Aside from that, motels, fetish clubs, or a dark corner of a gay bar can be exciting.

"Anyplace, but not too risky. Bedroom is best, but rest areas can be hot."

"The bedroom, however, I find it stimulating to almost be caught by others nearby."

"Any room in the house . . . anywhere I can lie down."

WHAT PUTS YOU IN THE MOOD FOR SEX?

Virgo is a visually oriented Sign. It's easy to put him in the mood for sex. Watching porn, the sight of his lover's nude body, or seeing an attractive man on the street is all that is necessary.

"All it takes is a gentle touch or seeing someone who I find attractive."

"Damn near anything. Just the sight of a nude or semi-nude man is enough for me."

"I can be put in the mood in a matter of seconds, mostly by touch."

"Showering/cleanliness, light, nice scent, watching porn, being touched, getting my partner turned on."

WHAT'S YOUR ATTITUDE TOWARD PORNOGRAPHY?

Virgo is likely to own a large collection of pornography. Even if he says it's not really his thing, Virgo uses it for self-satisfaction.

"It's great to watch while exercising on my stationary bike. Beats boredom."

"Mixed feelings, I enjoy it as a supplement to my sex life, but I fear that it has the potential to detract from true intimacy with my partner. I also worry that it causes sort of an alienation where a person retreats into their fantasies rather than experience the physical."

"It serves a useful purpose, ideal for foreplay or self-satisfaction."

MEMORIES

"Years ago I was in Central Park in NYC, in a cruising area. I was standing up against a rock with my pants down, just letting anyone who so desired suck my cock. Six or eight guys did so. I think about it often."

"I hired a hustler. He was a body builder with really big muscles. He had a huge muscular ass, with a very deep crack. After I licked his ass and sucked his big cock and his low hanging nuts, I fucked his ass intensely. I definitely got my money's worth."

HOW MUCH CUDDLING DO YOU ENJOY, ASIDE FROM SEX?

Virgo loves to cuddle, especially in private. When he's out in public he doesn't like his partner to be draped on him.

HOW TACTILE AND HOW ORAL ARE YOU?

Virgo is among the most tactile lovers in the zodiac, and he has few reservations about oral sex, though not all Virgos enjoy rimming.

"I have my hands over my lover's body from start to finish."

A MEMORY

"One summer, home from college I was staying with my sister. My boyfriend lived with his parents. We were having trouble finding time alone. Finally, after being interrupted for the umpteenth time, we went for a drive. We pulled off the road into a secluded area and parked. I kicked off my shoes and socks, pulled off my jeans and underwear, and climbed into the back seat. I lay there on my back with my legs spread and stroked my dick a few times.

"My boyfriend took off all of his clothes and climbed on top of me. With a little bit of spit he lubed up and slid inside me. He fucked me for about 15 minutes like that. He kept pausing to get 'comfortable.' What he was really doing was prolonging the whole thing. My legs were hurting, my ass was sore from the pounding and my dick was turning purple from being teased by his stomach hair. I told him I couldn't take any more so he came, then swooped down to suck me off. After two pumps with his mouth I unloaded a record amount of sperm into him."

"I absolutely love touch. I could spend hours exploring my lover's body with just my fingertips."

"Feeling him up gets us both hot."

"I love rimming ass holes. Rimming is really hot and can make me shoot just licking a guy's ass."

"I want to consume my lover, taking as much of him into my mouth as possible. I love to kiss him and lick every square inch of his body."

"I am very oral, I think giving head to a guy is one of the sexiest things in the world."

WHAT SEX ACTS DO YOU LIKE MOST AND LEAST?

He enjoys the entire range of mainstream sexual expression, from cuddling and kissing to oral and anal sex.

"In order of preference: kissing, receiving oral sex, giving oral sex, penetrative anal, receptive anal.

"For me, giving oral sex comes first. Receiving anal sex is in second place."

The more open Virgo adds:

"Nipple play, rimming, both giving and receiving, shaving, and enemas."

Virgo generally dislikes rough sex.

"I dislike extreme fetishes, such as fisting, water sports, extreme pain."

AS A LOVER, WHAT'S YOUR BEST SKILL?

Virgo is the Sign of work. He works hard at all things, including satisfying his partner sexually.

"I really think I give good head. My goal is to see how hard I can make him cum. I can use my tongue and the inner walls of my cheeks quite well while I suck."

"My hands—for his back, body, cock; my tongue—for licking his body all over; and my mouth to take his cock."

"I give a hell of a blow job. I fuck well, too."

WHAT SMELLS AND TASTES ON YOUR PARTNER DO YOU ENJOY?

He loves the smell of his partner's skin and mild cologne. He also enjoys the taste of pre-cum and clean fresh skin.

"Clean skin, sweat smell from having foreplay, sometimes underarms."

"Light body odor is okay but not strong perspiration, I like the smell of his cock and balls."

"Very slightly sweaty smell around the groin."

"I think that first taste of an erection is heavenly."

"I prefer just out of the shower or a very slight sweaty taste on the penis."

FOR SOME PEOPLE THE TASTE OF THEIR PARTNER'S CUM IS UNPLEASANT. IF THAT'S TRUE FOR YOU, WHAT DO YOU DO ABOUT THE TASTE?

He has little problem with the taste of his partner's cum. If it bothers him, he finds ways to handle it, for example by keeping something to drink beside the bed.

"I like the taste. I'll swallow, I'll take it on my face, I'll take it anywhere on or in my body."

"I think the taste is great. I am a swallower. The feeling of his orgasm down my throat is a major turn-on for me."

"I enjoy the sensation, not specifically the taste and swallow with monogamous partners only."

"I have the guy blow his load right down the back of my throat. I guzzle it right down. I do find the taste of most men's cum unpleasant."

"I wash it down with soda."

A MEMORY

"On a cross country trip a few years ago, I looked up an old high school friend. We had huge crushes on each other back then. We went over to his apartment. He began showing me photos of himself. We were sitting on his bed. The sexual tension was high. Within twenty minutes he was kissing me and we were ripping each other's clothes off. It felt as though we had unfinished business from all those years ago because we'd never had sex.

"We went at each other aggressively. I fucked him in every position possible, enraptured by a long-standing desire, and taken over by the intense feeling of skin to skin contact I had not previously experienced. He was wilder and more vocal than anyone I had fucked previously, biting his pillow many times to keep from screaming out loud. I came all over him."

"The taste doesn't bother me, but generally I let it drip out of my mouth onto his chest."

DO YOU ENJOY WATCHING YOUR PARTNER DURING SEX AND ORGASM? DO YOU ENJOY BEING WATCHED?

As this is a man who often enjoys ménage à trois, exhibitionism, and watching pornography, looking at his partner is a vital part of his sexual pleasure as is being watched by him.

"I really love watching a big load shoot."

"His facial expressions are wonderful."

The Big "O"

HOW DO YOU REACH AN ORGASM AND HOW OFTEN?

Virgo enjoys a range of stimulation to achieve orgasm. Most often he climaxes though masturbation, and he has an orgasm every time he has sex.

"I usually have to jerk myself off to finish things, very rarely ejaculate any other way."

"Mostly through masturbation but I prefer to do it by fucking a nice ass."

WHAT'S YOUR FAVORITE POSITION?

He likes virtually every position with some preference to straddle his lover.

"I am on top sitting on his penis. That way I am in control of the sex."

"Sitting on my lover's cock, while he is on his back, doggie style too."

"Orally, while I am lying on my back, but standing up is okay."

"Lying on my back with my mouth on someone's dick, butt, or mouth."

"I like '69.' Once we find a rhythm '69' is the best way to achieve simultaneous orgasm."

SOME PEOPLE ARE CONCERNED ABOUT BRINGING A PARTNER TO CLIMAX BEFORE HAVING AN ORGASM THEMSELVES. OTHERS STRIVE TO REACH ORGASM TOGETHER. WHICH IS TRUE FOR YOU?

He prefers to climax with his partner and, given Virgo's systematic approach to sex, an orderly process from A to B to C then on to O, he is usually successful in accomplishing it.

"Cumming at the same time is best."

"Try to do it together most times, other times try to bring him to climax before I cum."

"I prefer to reach it together, absolutely hate it if one person is left out."

ARE YOU VOCAL DURING SEX?

Though he makes his likes and dislikes clearly known, he does this more often before having sex. In other words, he will talk abut sex openly with a potential partner but during the act he is only moderately vocal.

AFTER SEX WHAT DO YOU LIKE TO DO?

Whatever else he might want to do, he'll want to shower after sex, and any post-sex activity will be quiet.

"Shower and then spend time together, regardless of activity."

"It depends on the situation, usually fall off to sleep together."

"Just lie there holding each other."

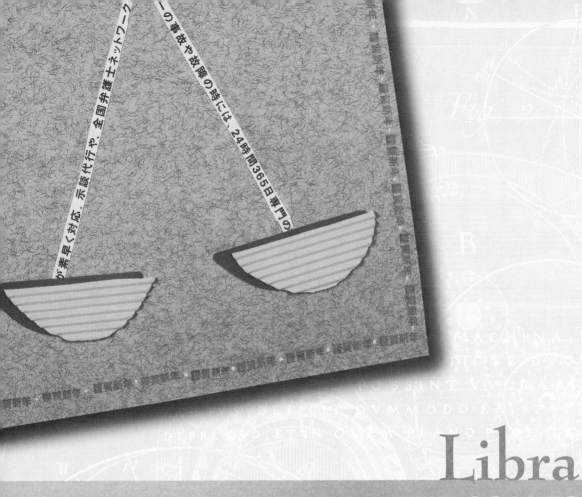

Libra
THE SCALES
September 23 through October 22

AIR SIGN LIBRA, romantic, good-natured, and courteous, strives for harmony, and hates discord. The Sign of commitment and partnership, Libras find fulfillment through their relationships. Ruler of the kidneys, loins, and lower back, a sensual massage and attention to the backside add to their sexual pleasure.

What he says: "I love to touch, especially the feel of a guy's ass in my hands, even in a sensual spanking."

"In love the paradox occurs that two beings become one and yet remain two."
—Erich Fromm

The Libra Man
in His Own Words

A MEMORY

"There was a man I had wanted to be with for some time. He kept putting me off. It drove me crazy. One day he let me have a shot at him in a parked van on a dead-end street. We lit a flashlight. He dropped his jeans, and let me admire him front and back. What surprised me was that he unzipped me, fished it out, and really went all out to satisfy me. I told him that I needed to taste him. It was the first time I really cared about the other guy enjoying himself. We got into frottage, which I love. It was awkward for him. He wasn't into this. He did this to make a moment for me. When I realized his power, I let one of my best orgasms rip. I still remember his masculine voice, his hairy body, and the sounds of him slurping on my cock."

Attraction and Dating a Libra

WHAT ATTRACTS YOU TO SOMEONE?

Libra is the Sign of beauty and attracting a Libra's attention requires both nice features and a fit physique. Libra also hates discord, so a man who is genial and even-tempered is a natural match for him.

"I notice a man's face, the size of his arms, chest, and waist and then the texture of his hair."

"First of all, quite good looking, then funny and who likes me for me and not just for sex, someone who is outgoing and not too queeny."

"I am always taken by nice lips, teeth and eyes and facial hair. I like beefy stocky men that tend to be straight acting."

"People with beautiful eyes, nice bodies, not over developed, and sweet and sunny personalities, always attract me."

WHAT MIGHT TURN YOU OFF?

Libra is a well-mannered individual who cares about relating well to others. Therefore, unpleasant behavior in public, little attention to hygiene, or being out of shape turn him off.

"A man who is rude or disrespectful of himself or others turns me off."

"Someone who is too fat or too thin and doesn't take care of himself."

"A man who is insincere or unkind won't interest me."

A FANTASY

"I often jack off with guys on the Internet, both by verbal method and on camera. As I am writing this I am excited by the thought of some stranger's cock jacking with mine, cumming. I love to watch them cum. I have a great cock for the camera, and most guys love to watch me jack off too. Sometimes I fantasize about a third person along with my partner and me."

WHAT DO YOU ENJOY DOING ON A DATE?

Libra likes to go out, to be treated as someone special. He wants time to talk and then enjoys going on to an activity such as seeing a movie or even taking a walk. Overall, he prefers evenings out, rather than staying in. Dining out, even at a casual café, is preferable to cooking a meal at home.

"Going to the theater, a movie, a restaurant, taking long walks, sitting and talking."

"Pleasant conversation, usually something active like physical exercise."

"Drinks, dinner, and a movie, walking through the streets of New York on a Sunday afternoon."

"I enjoy talking, going out to eat or a movie, then if he is into it, we make out."

ARE YOU FLIRTATIOUS?

Libra is an Air Sign at ease conversing with anyone. His genial nature makes him a charming flirt.

"I enjoy engaging attractive people in conversation, which may be construed as flirtatious, but it is not my intention to get them to have sex."

"Yes and much more so when I know it's a safe environment."

"I am known as a constant flirt."

ARE YOU JEALOUS?

To the extent that anyone can be jealous on occasion, he is, but jealousy is not a significant problem for Libra.

"I would say, somewhat, not overly."

"No, I sometimes feel a pang of jealousy, but it usually passes quickly; we all need space."

HOW DO YOU FEEL ABOUT PUBLIC DISPLAYS OF AFFECTION?

Libra's only hesitation on this subject concerns personal safety. In such places as Provincetown, Fort Lauderdale, and San Francisco he enjoys being openly demonstrative.

"I would love to show public affection, but where I live that would be unacceptable."

"More power to you . . . excellent fun."

"I encourage and welcome it. . . . It is great."

"I love it, but do it in a respectful manner."

A MEMORY

"It was three years ago. I was at a group meeting, disinterested, and bored. I wanted to leave as soon as I got there and then this kid arrived, about twenty-four years old. I had never felt this way before. His small hands, smooth as silk, his face with a quiet smile. A friend got us together. Then that weekend we met. We parked the car, kissed. I felt his face with my eyes closed. I remember thinking, 'This can't be true, it is like a dream come true.' We went to his place. He showed me to his bedroom and I let him take over."

Sexual Attitudes and Behaviors

HOW OFTEN DO YOU THINK ABOUT SEX AND HOW OFTEN PER WEEK DO YOU WANT TO HAVE SEX?

He is not preoccupied with sex, though he thinks about it often, and when he is with a partner who matches his sex drive, he enjoys having sex on a daily basis. At the least, he wants to have sex three times per week.

"Every day, but I keep it to three times a week . . . otherwise I would never get any work done."

"I enjoy having sex daily when my partner is staying with me."

HOW LONG DO YOU LIKE TO SPEND HAVING SEX AND HOW MUCH OF THAT TIME IS FOREPLAY? DO YOU ENJOY QUICKIES?

Libra prefers to take his time having sex, with the average being forty-five minutes to an hour per session, half of which is foreplay. Sometimes he enjoys longer sessions. Quickies are not his favorite things.

"I spend as much time as possible having sex. I don't enjoy quickies."

"The more time the better. I strive for endurance, and foreplay really enhances the experience. As to quickies, unless I've been with the same partner a while, they don't interest me."

"The amount of time I spend on foreplay varies, but I like to move slowly into things."

WHAT TIME OF DAY DO YOU PREFER TO HAVE SEX?

Libra is available any time of day or night with some preference for daylight hours, from early morning right through the evening.

"Anytime. When I am involved with someone I usually do it in the morning."

"I am a guy! I'll take it whenever I can get the time to have it."

"I am an afternoon person, but anytime works for a quickie."

HOW OFTEN PER WEEK DO YOU MASTURBATE?

He masturbates two to four times a week.

HOW LONG DO YOU WANT TO KNOW SOMEONE BEFORE GETTING SEXUAL?

On average he hopes to become sexual with a new partner on the second date. However, experience has taught him that getting to know a man for a while, before sex becomes part of the relationship, works out better for long-term involvement.

"Touching and kissing begins immediately, more sexual behavior happens as things progress."

"Depends on the person and the circumstance, sometimes, right upon meeting, other times, wait until we are dating."

"I usually want to have sex right away, if a guy is my type. However, this has not led to a real ongoing connection of any length."

> **A FANTASY**
>
> "When I am alone in bed I have this fantasy about sex with a young man, kissing him all over, and letting him do me as he pleases, then I get to suck his cock until he is bone dry. I want to have intercourse but can't because I am too big to fit in him, so I let him sit on top of me so I can feel every part of his small body."

WHAT'S YOUR ATTITUDE TOWARD CASUAL SEX?

He realizes he should take his time and is known to debate things long and hard before acting, but when he meets an appealing and willing man he is likely to engage in anonymous sex.

"I see nothing wrong with casual sex if you're single."

"It is fine. I make no judgment about it. I have participated in it. It serves its purpose."

"Fine, I think it is okay when you are safe."

DO YOU BELIEVE IN MONOGAMY?

He does believe in the concept of monogamy but may not practice it. Libra's behavior in a relationship is highly contingent upon the desires of his partner. In other words, he will be monogamous if his lover prefers that arrangement. He will welcome other lovers if that is not a problem.

"Yes, for those who are willing and capable of making that commitment. I know it's not for everyone."

"I believe in monogamy but feel it's very difficult to find others who do."

"Yes, I do, even though it is rare. I believe that two men can fully satisfy each other."

A MEMORY

"Waking up on a rainy morning in Hawaii. The smell of the rain and the scent of my lover made my cock hard. Because of the warmth, my balls were hanging low. My lover was sleeping as my hard cock was pressed against his side. He stirred. I felt his nipples and they hardened, smelled his underarms and started licking from there to his nipple. I sucked his nipple, pressed my cock against his side. His cock was now standing straight up so I went right down on it with my mouth, taking it all down my throat. He grabbed my cock and started jacking it, as I sucked and he fucked my face. Shortly he exploded in my mouth and I came all over his body. UMM."

DOES SEX HAVE A SPIRITUAL SIGNIFICANCE FOR YOU?

Libra enjoys casual sex yet also believes in monogamy. Spirituality depends on the nature of the relationship.

"Sex can be a transcendent experience, leading to transformation, when it's really good."

"Yes, in giving a part of me to my partner."

"When I enter into sexual intimacy I acknowledge that I am experiencing another embodiment of the divine."

"With my partner, yes. It feels as if we are making love and taking our love to another level. Sex with us has only gotten better over the years, the more spiritual we grow."

ARE YOU COMFORTABLE INITIATING SEXUAL ACTIVITIES?

Libra has no trouble being the initiator, but he might hold back because he doesn't want to make anyone uncomfortable. The fact is that he has a strong sex drive and is receptive to a man's sexual advances most of the time, so he prefers that a partner do the initiating.

HOW DO YOU COMMUNICATE TO YOUR PARTNER YOUR SEXUAL WANTS AND NEEDS?

Libra is an Air Sign, a Sign of communication. Once comfortable in a relationship he is at ease in letting his partner know how to please him, and he appreciates a man telling him what feels good as well.

"Usually by talking beforehand. During foreplay it is all gestures and symbols."

"Both words and gestures, open communication, exploration, and humor."

"Most often with gestures, only words when absolutely necessary. How I respond to my partner's touches lets him know what I like."

DO YOU THINK OF YOURSELF AS BEING IN THE MAINSTREAM SEXUALLY, MORE EXPERIMENTAL, OR OPEN TO ANYTHING?

His range of sexuality goes from mainstream to experimental. He is likely to engage in anal sex, bondage, exhibitionism, sex in public places, and voyeurism. Provocative underwear turns him on as does using food along with sex. Libra likes pastry, sweet foods, and whipped cream. He may also enjoy a ménage à trois or an orgy. When it comes to sex toys he uses dildoes and vibrators, cock rings, and occasionally bondage items.

Libra's fantasies usually incorporate scenes of oral and anal sex and other mainstream activities that he is likely to engage in with a partner.

HOW DO YOU DEMONSTRATE AFFECTION FOR YOUR PARTNER?

Reflecting his nature both as an Air Sign and the Sign of relationships, Libra is thoughtful and caring and shows his regard most consistently by listening to his partner.

"Most of all I listen, and also by touching, making food, assisting and sharing tasks, saying 'I love you,' and spontaneous kissing."

"By listening to his day, cuddling, doing things for him when he comes home."

"I leave him little notes, tokens of my regard, and by paying special attention to him."

FANTASIES

"A delicious flavored substance put all over the body, in a form of a trail and turn off the lights and use my tongue from the start point to the end. And maybe start all over again."

"I fantasize about great threesomes and orgies and sometimes about rough sex, where I am lightly punched on both sides of the head while I am performing oral sex."

The Five Senses

● ●

HOW IMPORTANT TO YOU IS THE SEXUAL ENVIRONMENT?

While the person he's with matters more than the location, Libra is romantic and a clean, pleasant setting will enhance the experience for him. An exception is the occasional spontaneous quickie.

A MEMORY

"It was a summer afternoon, about seventy-five to eighty degrees, at a gay nudist compound in the Pocono Mountains. My partner and I were listening to a Miles Davis kind of blues album, sitting outside his tent when this hot body builder came over to join us. We talked for a few minutes and it became obvious that we were all interested in sex. I knelt in front of the body builder and went down on him. He smelled slightly of sweat and tasted salty. Then the three of us went inside for privacy. It was remarkably comfortable for all of us."

"Cleanliness counts. I hate a dirty place or bed."

"I prefer cleanliness, candles, and soft music."

"The person means more than the environment, unless it is straight out sleazy and unsanitary."

"The environment is key, it must be comfortable, not distracting."

WHERE DO YOU LIKE TO HAVE SEX?

Libra is not terribly adventurous. He prefers having sex in the bedroom as it meets his criteria: clean, comfortable, and safe.

"Preferably the bedroom, but anyplace is fine with the right person."

"Indoors, anywhere, secluded outdoors spots."

"Any place that is comfortable, usually in the bedroom."

WHAT PUTS YOU IN THE MOOD FOR SEX?

Air Sign Libra is turned on by words. Sexy conversation and pornography put him in the mood. Sensual places, such as dimly lit clubs or the beach at night, also get him primed.

"Good conversation and good wine, smells, natural, not cologne, temperature is important. I lose it in the cold . . . below sixty degrees Fahrenheit."

"Showering, watching and reading porn, as well as being rested."

"Music, nature of the environment (gay club), and when I'm alone watching porn, especially two or more guys having wild sex."

WHAT'S YOUR ATTITUDE TOWARD PORNOGRAPHY?

Libra strives to get along with people, seeking balance in his relationships. Regarding pornography, he likes to use it when he is alone. He doesn't use it with a partner until he knows how his lover feels about porn.

"I love the visuals of pornography as a means of providing arousal."

"Sometimes it is fun, like cotton candy . . . sweet, but not much substance."

"I enjoy pornography, an occasional film, and magazines with hot photos and good info."

"It's fine as a masturbation aide, but I find it distracting from intimacy when I am with a partner."

A MEMORY

"Sex with an ex who was a muscular carpenter and used no colognes or deodorants, but was squeaky clean. We kissed, caressed, had oral and anal sex for hours at a time. His masculine aromas and hard body were a turn-on. We usually fell asleep afterwards in each other's arms."

HOW MUCH CUDDLING DO YOU ENJOY, ASIDE FROM SEX?

He may not want a man to hang all over him, but as long as the location is gay friendly, Libra says, "Bring on the cuddling."

"Cuddling is a major part of a relationship, with or without sex."

"Lots, with some one I am attracted to, otherwise, please don't touch me."

"Lots, almost more than sex."

"Cuddling is great, with the exception of when I am trying to sleep, then I want my own space."

HOW TACTILE AND HOW ORAL ARE YOU?

Libra is very into touch and oral sex. He may love or hate rimming but otherwise there's no limit to his oral play.

"I am highly tactile and love to explore with my hands. I am equally oral, love deep kissing and giving him head."

"I love to touch, especially the feel of a guy's ass in my hand, even in a sensual spanking. I love deep mouth kissing, rimming too, and I also enjoy sucking on a big cock."

"Touching—a lot, from head to toe. I enjoy oral anywhere on the body, but no rimming."

"I love to touch and be touched all over as well as kissing and licking his body and sucking nipples."

FANTASIES

"They include scenarios from raunchy to the sublime, all intensely pleasurable, such as a bareback, fisting party, with lots of hairy, muscle pigs, riding the range or highways with cowboys, or a motorcycle club and servicing the gang as a virtual fuck hole."

"Having an experience of being dominated and my partner being verbally aggressive, not abusive, but making me surrender to him, really taking control of me."

WHAT SEX ACTS DO YOU LIKE MOST AND LEAST?

There's little he doesn't like in the mainstream range of sex, though anal is his least favorite act, and it is rare for Libra to experiment with any sex acts having to do with dominance, submission, humiliation, or sadomasochism.

"My favorites are kissing, oral sex, and mutual masturbation."

"I enjoy oral sex the most, but the rest is not far behind. I don't like anything that causes injury or is unsafe."

"Love kissing, hugging, frottage, nipple play, fellatio, rimming, fucking, getting fucked, and fisting. I don't like cock and ball torture or sensory deprivation."

"I love sucking cock, being sucked, kissing, frottage, mutual masturbation, and rubbing our cocks together."

AS A LOVER, WHAT'S YOUR BEST SKILL?

Libra, as the Sign of relationships, strives to satisfy his lover by extending himself, responding to his partner, kissing with great feeling, touching with sensitivity.

"How I read my partner's desires. I always know what is going on in his head. Old boyfriends have wanted to end the relationship but not the sex."

"I have extremely healing hands and a way of looking into my lover's eyes that intensify the experience. I also use my breath as a sexual organ."

"My childlike curiosity to explore and be the best, especially with my tongue, hands, and body."

"My mouth and hands are constant explorers, but my cock is king."

WHAT SMELLS AND TASTES ON YOUR PARTNER DO YOU ENJOY?

Libra is quite sensual. The smells and tastes of his lover's skin, all over the body, from his neck to his groin, please him most when unadorned by colognes.

"I enjoy smelling his manly body odors, not talking raunch, smelling his jock and ass hole. The taste of a man's lips is the ultimate, but I also enjoy the taste of a guy's cock and I really get into licking, sucking, and nibbling a guy's nice buns."

"A hint of the smell of natural body odor, a hint of salty taste from sweat is best."

"Underarms, his body odor when he gets excited, his feet, and ear lobes. The taste of his nipples, balls, feet, ears, just about all of it."

"The smell of skin, armpits, crotch, ass. As to tastes, everything, if he is clean."

A FANTASY

"My fantasies include living in an ashram as an ascetic practicing tantric sex or candaulism, watching a couple engage in sex. In another fantasy I imagine that I am living in nature among a colony of fellow nudists, practicing Native American sexual rites and assuming roles as animals."

FOR SOME PEOPLE THE TASTE OF THEIR PARTNER'S CUM IS UNPLEASANT. IF THAT'S TRUE FOR YOU, WHAT DO YOU DO ABOUT THE TASTE?

Libra revels in the taste and smell of cum.

"I love his cum, all of it, taste and smell. I eat it and rub it on my face and body."

"The taste of his cum is a real turn-on. I swallow or we rub it on each other."

"I love the taste of cum. I swallow or rub it on him. I fall asleep at night tasting it."

MEMORIES

"Dinner, a long conversation slowly turning into touching and then sex."

"A quickie with a stranger in a large heated pool."

"Making love on a bed covered with rose petals."

"He was totally into me. We made out, fucked and fingered, spanked, used bondage. Throughout he was always touching me."

DO YOU ENJOY WATCHING YOUR PARTNER DURING SEX AND ORGASM? DO YOU ENJOY BEING WATCHED?

Yes, to both. One of the traits of Libra is striving to live life to the fullest. In his sexual relations this means satisfying all his senses, touch, smell, taste, and sight too.

"Watching, oh yes, very much, and being watched, even more so. I am an exhibitionist. I love to show off."

"It's all fine and, yes, I enjoy him watching me."

"I love to watch my guy during the whole sexual experience and orgasm. The idea of being watched is appealing, but I am not that comfortable with it yet."

The Big "O"

HOW DO YOU REACH AN ORGASM AND HOW OFTEN?

Libra has no difficulty achieving orgasm. He climaxes from oral sex, masturbation, anal sex, or a combination of these acts.

"A combination of sex acts . . . I enjoy being fingered anally, while my partner masturbates me."

"I always cum, sometimes while giving head or when I'm being jerked off."

WHAT'S YOUR FAVORITE POSITION?

He mentions liking them all, on top, on the bottom, facing side by side, "69." But his real preference is for doggie style.

SOME PEOPLE ARE CONCERNED ABOUT BRINGING A PARTNER TO CLIMAX BEFORE HAVING AN ORGASM THEMSELVES. OTHERS STRIVE TO REACH ORGASM TOGETHER. WHICH IS TRUE FOR YOU?

This is not an issue of consequence for Libra. He wants his partner to make an effort to put him in the mood with sexy talk, but once things get going he likes to please his partner. Seeing his lover satisfied matters more than who comes first or getting there at the same time.

"We like to cum together, but often he cums first."

"Mutual orgasm is the best. Otherwise I prefer bringing my partner to climax, then I get off."

"It would be ultimate to reach orgasm simultaneously. This happens rarely. When I am really into a guy I want him to experience a climax more."

"This is not an issue. I couldn't care less as long as we both climax."

"I'm not overly concerned with it either way; however it manifests is perfect."

ARE YOU VOCAL DURING SEX?

Considering that Libra is an Air Sign, it may seem surprising but he is not very vocal during sex. Only after he knows a man quite well does he relax and allow himself to express his responses openly.

AFTER SEX WHAT DO YOU LIKE TO DO?

He doesn't like to rush and personal appearance is important to him, so it isn't often that he will want to go out after sex, unless there's plenty of time to shower and get ready.

"Take a nap, then go again."

"Shower with him, then cuddle."

"I prefer sharing a shower, holding hands, hugging, and letting him know how much the sex together affected me."

A MEMORY

"My lover and I rented a cabin at a mountain resort for a weekend one summer. The days were warm, the nights chilly. We had a wonderful fireplace and were very comfortable, so much so that we spent the whole weekend nude, except for boots and backpacks. We had sex everywhere, meeting other men and having sex spontaneously. We had an orgy at our cabin and twenty to twenty-five men came and went through the night and into the next day."

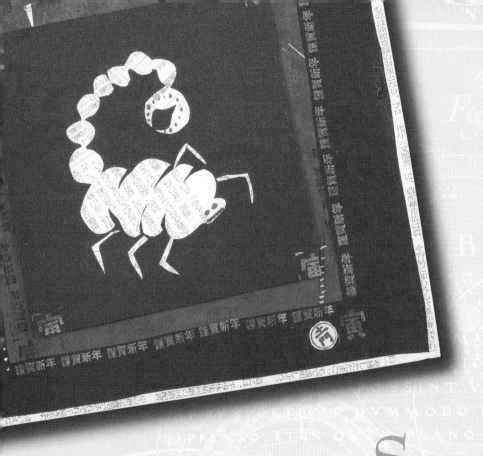

Scorpio
THE SCORPION
October 23 through November 21

WATER SIGN SCORPIO is powerful, emotional, intense, and secretive. Ruler of the genitals, Scorpio is the Sign of sex. Rushing to the heart of the matter, his penis, will turn off Scorpio. Some teasing and build up makes the experience far more passionate for this Sign.

What he says: "I have made my partners cum in their pants with just my tongue and hands."

"[Sex is] the most fun I have ever had without laughing."

—Woody Allen,
screenplay for Annie Hall

The Scorpio Man in His Own Words

"I was assisting a customer in the dressing room of the store I managed. He decided I needed to give him head. His hot, hard cock was pure heaven, clean, fresh smelling. The thought of getting caught was a serious adrenaline rush."

Attraction and Dating a Scorpio

WHAT ATTRACTS YOU TO SOMEONE?

A man's physique may first attract Scorpio, but it is his energy and general behavior that will hold Scorpio's attention. He wants a man to be focused completely on him. Eyes that wander around the room will undermine Scorpio's interest. In fact, eye contact is of great importance in developing a relationship with him. Scorpio cares about penis size. Perhaps enormous is not necessary; impressive will do.

"Penis size counts with me, hair, physique, weight, beauty, energy, funny, smart, goal oriented, family oriented, nurturing, clean, no drugs, as little baggage as possible."

"The first thing I notice about a man is his smile. Then I look for a spark in the eyes, attentiveness, and caring."

"A man who is comfortable within himself, romantic, down to earth, an equal partner."

"I think it is a combination of factors . . . hairy chest, nice eyes, being in shape and fit. Personality is important, as well as being upbeat, sensitive, and passionate."

"A good attitude and nice smile attract me to someone."

"I respond to a man that is older, mature, real, who makes eye contact, and doesn't have an attitude. Looks are unimportant."

WHAT MIGHT TURN YOU OFF?

Scorpio prefers men who look somewhat conservative and sedate as opposed to the man with copious piercings and spiked hair.

"Turn-offs: conceit, negative energy towards other people, lack of self-respect."

"Bizarre appearance and behavior, lack of personal hygiene, and fat."

"Someone who is insecure, feminine acting, uses drugs or smokes, drinks excessively, or thinks he is God's gift to homosexuality."

"A bad attitude or someone who talks only about himself turns me off more than any particular physical attribute. Of course, he shouldn't be dirty or unkempt."

MEMORIES

"My lover and I had sex at a rest area while a hot leather man watched. I went down on my lover while the guy masturbated himself. It was intimidating and exciting at the same time."

"A guy who was primarily straight, wore fingerless gloves (my fetish), and the sex lasted for hours."

WHAT DO YOU ENJOY DOING ON A DATE?

Scorpio is an intense person, bored with superficiality and trivial conversation. On an evening out he wants a chance to get to know a man in some depth. Even with a long-term partner he prefers thoughtful conversation.

"Hanging out with my friends to see if he fits in, playing video games, and watching TV."

"On a first date, the most important thing is being able to communicate."

"Dinner and conversation is always a good thing. Going out for coffee is another way that I like to break the ice, if I don't want to be committed to a dinner situation."

"I enjoy going out to dinner and participating in outdoor activities in which I can still interact with the other person. In other words, a movie is a bad date to me."

"Food, a passion of mine, either dinner out or homemade, conversation, exploring interests, humor."

ARE YOU FLIRTATIOUS?

He is flirtatious only in a very quiet way, more in the way that he looks at a man rather than by overt gesture or with a direct approach.

"Yes, but subtly, especially when I am really attracted to someone."

"I would say that I am not really flirtatious, just friendly."

"Yes, no doubt, I am flirty. If someone shows interest I usually play along with it, but I am always honest with people and do not lead anyone on in a negative way."

ARE YOU JEALOUS?

Scorpio, as a Sign, has the reputation for being quite jealous but he does not see himself that way. Well, he will admit to being somewhat jealous, especially if the man he is with responds to another person's flirtation.

"If I am attracted to someone I can get very jealous."

"Sometimes, but not often. Isn't everyone a little?"

"Yes, I need to admit that I can be jealous at times."

"Not often, and getting better about it."

HOW DO YOU FEEL ABOUT PUBLIC DISPLAYS OF AFFECTION?

Scorpio is a secretive Sign. He is decidedly uncomfortable with almost any public displays of affection.

"I am not interested. I do not want to see it and I'm not into showing."

"Beyond handholding and hugging, it makes me feel very uneasy."

"A little is okay in a gay environment, but I am not big on public displays of affection."

A FANTASY

"I imagine having sex on a private beach, just before the sun goes down, at the end of a hot day. I hear the waves crashing in the background and alternative music playing. We are sweating, allowing our oiled bodies to slide and rub gently without friction, and then we take turns sucking and fucking."

Sexual Attitudes and Behaviors

. . . .

HOW OFTEN DO YOU THINK ABOUT SEX AND HOW OFTEN PER WEEK DO YOU WANT TO HAVE SEX?

Whether he wants more or less sex is dependent upon the emotional interaction with his partner. Scorpio, the Sign of sex, in general, enjoys having sex four times per week.

"I can go without sex for weeks, then want it every day."

"If I could, all the time."

HOW LONG DO YOU LIKE TO SPEND HAVING SEX AND HOW MUCH OF THAT TIME IS FOREPLAY? DO YOU ENJOY QUICKIES?

Scorpio prefers taking his time at sex so he is not overly enthusiastic about quickies. He prefers keeping foreplay fairly short, five to ten minutes, with the maximum being a half hour.

"I like to spend a half hour to an hour all together for sex. No, I do not like quickies."

"An hour, up to ninety minutes, and no to quickies."

"How much time depends on circumstances. Generally one half to a full hour, and yes, quickies are okay as well."

"Yes, I enjoy quickies though not as a steady diet."

"I don't really enjoy quickies, but I do them every once in a great while."

"Let's get on with the show. I don't mind a little foreplay but I don't want to spend more than ten to fifteen minutes on it."

"I like sex for an hour. Foreplay is about 70 percent of sex."

WHAT TIME OF DAY DO YOU PREFER TO HAVE SEX?

He's happy to have sex virtually at any time of day or night.

"Anytime is wonderful, but my favorite is right after waking up in the morning."

"Sex is great all day, anytime, but I do love morning."

HOW OFTEN PER WEEK DO YOU MASTURBATE?

Scorpio is a very sexual Sign. Even when having an active sex life with a partner he is likely to masturbate three to five times weekly.

HOW LONG DO YOU WANT TO KNOW SOMEONE BEFORE GETTING SEXUAL?

When he becomes sexual with a man upon a first encounter, in all likelihood the interaction will be merely casual sex. Scorpio is a man of depth. A true relationship grows out of mutual interests and a strong sense of connection. As a result, time is a variable, dependent upon the nature of the developing relationship.

"That depends on the person. If I am interested in his intellect it could be a long time. If it's just about sex, that same night."

"The amount of time is determined by how long it takes me to be fully comfortable with a man."

"It varies, but in a potential relationship situation, I would rather wait a few dates."

"Depends on the person, I have been sexual on the first date and other times not at all."

A FANTASY

"A romantic encounter, dim lights— just enough to see him, following a night of dancing, where he has a slight odor from his groin and feet, not strong. I start by taking his clothes off and kissing and massaging his feet and work my way up his body, stopping at his groin, ass, nipples, armpits, ears, and mouth. He would then enter me and climax, after which I would do the same to him."

WHAT'S YOUR ATTITUDE TOWARD CASUAL SEX?

Scorpio is somewhat conflicted about casual sex. On the one hand, he regards it as unsafe or even immoral. Nevertheless he enjoys it and is apt to be a player.

"As long as all parties involved know the line between love and sex, I truly enjoy it."

"It is unsafe, but fun."

"I think it is immoral, but I have done it anyway. In fact, enjoyed it."

"It is fine if both people are into it and want to do it."

DO YOU BELIEVE IN MONOGAMY?

Scorpio is a fixed Sign meaning that he wants to be in a settled situation. He likes the stability and reliability of monogamy.

A MEMORY

"Hot sex. . . . You know it was hot when you shoot across the room. Sometimes it is fucking until your balls slap or a gentle stroking or petting of my cock can make me cum."

"In a committed relationship, monogamy is the ultimate compliment that two people can share. It shows complete intimacy with each other."

"Yes, if in a relationship sex should only be with that person."

"I feel that monogamy is a key ingredient in a successful relationship."

"Yes, but my partner and I play together with others."

DOES SEX HAVE A SPIRITUAL SIGNIFICANCE FOR YOU?

When he says to a man, "I love you," he means that he senses a connection, a bond that he feels deeply, something that touches that very lonely place in him. In such a relationship, sex is spiritual.

"Yes, because there is a huge difference between sex and fucking. Making love brings sex to a whole new level."

"Having sex with a person you love is very spiritual, it strengthens the bond between you."

"If love is involved, then sex is spiritual, otherwise it is animalistic satisfaction."

FANTASIES

"I envision being kidnapped and raped, obligated to have sex with my captor, kept tied up and forced to do what I am told."

"My fantasies are often about taboos: raping someone or incest-sex with my father. Other times I imagine someone worshiping my 10½ inch uncut thick cock."

ARE YOU COMFORTABLE INITIATING SEXUAL ACTIVITIES?

Given that Scorpio is the Sign of sex and has powerful magnetism, one might expect that he would always take the lead sexually. It's just not so. Scorpio is comfortable initiating sex only when he is confident that he will be well received.

"I would say that I am somewhat comfortable with this. If I am really in the mood I will initiate."

HOW DO YOU COMMUNICATE TO YOUR PARTNER YOUR SEXUAL WANTS AND NEEDS?

Even though Scorpio is highly sexual, he is uncomfortable being too direct when talking about what pleases him, especially with a new partner. He truly hopes that the other will figure him out and Scorpio's body language is quite clear. If his partner pays attention, he will know exactly how to make the Scorpion happy.

"If a partner does not understand my gesture, then I will use words to clarify my desires."

"Communicating leads to total understanding and trust."

DO YOU THINK OF YOURSELF AS BEING IN THE MAINSTREAM SEXUALLY, MORE EXPERIMENTAL, OR OPEN TO ANYTHING?

He is a somewhat experimental lover who is open to anal sex, both giving and receiving, exhibitionism, and ménage à trois. Scorpio may also enjoy incorporating food in sexual behaviors, spanking, tattoos, underwear, and voyeurism. Hairy men turn him on. He does not usually delve into more extreme bondage, or sado-masochism or the use of many sex toys. Virtually all Scorpio men enjoy having sex in public places.

Most of his fantasies are simple and straightforward with settings that range from romantic to scenes in which he is submissive.

HOW DO YOU DEMONSTRATE AFFECTION FOR YOUR PARTNER?

He is romantic and demonstrates affection for his partner with loving touches, thoughtful acts and small gifts. In return, he loves receiving a token gift for no reason and finding notes in unexpected places.

"Some kind of physical contact, touching, holding hands, surprise phone calls, e-mail, messages, doing things for him without his knowledge."

FANTASIES

"I envision a lazy, sunny day at the beach, all warm and tanned, a shower, a nap, and hours of licking, caressing, and fucking, with a man who knows how to do anal sex smoothly. That's all I need to think about."

"Very athletic guys being extremely physical with me."

"My fantasies usually involve multiple partners, orgies, also rhythmic anal sex, with smooth and steady undulations."

"A hot man in uniform, strips for me and pleases me long and hard. I am in my sexy underwear, a fetish of mine."

"Flowers, massages, leaving love notes and messages on the answer machine, doing his laundry."

"I do household chores for him and things he wouldn't expect, like ordering his favorite food without him even knowing I had called for take-out."

"I cook, I clean. I express my affection verbally as well as physically, as in a glance, a kiss, an embrace."

"I like to touch and kiss and also like to give massages."

The Five Senses

HOW IMPORTANT TO YOU IS THE SEXUAL ENVIRONMENT?

The environment for sex is of little importance to Scorpio. Satin sheets and candlelight might be wasted on him, and the setting does not have to be spotlessly clean.

"I like it to be clean, unless we're in a park where you can't help it. Dim light sets the mood for me."

"It's not important, dirty is even a bit sexy."

"Cleanliness is good but not critical."

"It is important to a point, but it is not a determining factor."

"The place should be clean."

A MEMORY

"I was approached in a dark corner of a sex club by three very handsome men. They proceeded to strip me down and each one was either kissing me, doing oral sex on me, or performing anal sex on me. It was dark, but I could see everything happening. The room smelled of sweaty men and bodily fluids. There were others watching and cheering us on."

WHERE DO YOU LIKE TO HAVE SEX?

Scorpio is a highly creative Sign, willing to have sex anywhere. In fact, a new lover, who wants to impress Scorpio, will suggest an unexpected and hidden setting for a sexual encounter.

"I have yet to find a place where I did not enjoy having sex."

"Everywhere, especially risky places."

"I am open to all places. Settings that are outside the norm, such as in cars, being outdoors, secluded but nonetheless in public, at a club, in a basement, out at a sex club all tend to make the sex more exciting."

WHAT PUTS YOU IN THE MOOD FOR SEX?

Scorpio is mysterious. Porn may do it today but not tomorrow. Feeling close and cuddling may work one day and not the next. Nothing in particular, everything in general, puts him in the mood.

"Just guys being guys or guys doing guy things, working out, mowing the lawn, watching sports."

"The interaction between my partner and me."

"Just plain desire for it."

"Phone sex with my partner."

"The person I am with, music, seeing him naked, porn, romantic activities."

"Candlelight, Cool Whip, spices, oils, jogging, showering, listening to Enigma, watching porn videos, hot tub, outside on a ninety-degree day with 100 percent humidity, ball massages."

WHAT'S YOUR ATTITUDE TOWARD PORNOGRAPHY?

Scorpio is of two minds on the subject of pornography, but whether he loves it or not, it does turn him on.

"I feel sorry for the participants in porn, but I do look at it to masturbate."

"I used to like it; now that I am in a relationship, I would rather tape us and watch it."

"I love it, especially since the Internet makes it so easily available."

A MEMORY

"I set up an entire day of sexual interludes. These encounters involved leaving notes and commands. We had a bubble bath, drank champagne, and used sex toys ranging from handcuffs to fire and oil. The scene was set with music in the background, candles, and flowers. We used lotions, gave each other massages. I had dirty pictures of myself. We started with slow dancing and proceeded to fucking and each of us had four orgasms that day."

HOW MUCH CUDDLING DO YOU ENJOY, ASIDE FROM SEX?

Scorpio enjoys a considerable amount of cuddling when spending quiet time with a partner, such as when watching TV. At other times, Scorpio wants his own space. He is a Water Sign, needing time for meditation.

"With someone I care about, when we have one on one time together, I like to cuddle as much as possible."

"I could do it all the time as long as he was holding me."

"I like to cuddle a little, I need my own space."

HOW TACTILE AND HOW ORAL ARE YOU?

Scorpio is the Sign of sex and enjoys exploring his lover's body equally with his hands and his mouth.

"I like to touch . . . his hands, chest, arms, and hair."

"I am very tactile. I love to feel my partner's body."

"Kissing is very, very important and I love to lick a firm chest and belly."

"I am very orally fixated. Kissing, blow jobs, my very favorite things."

"Kissing is okay. I do love giving blow jobs a lot, but rimming is gross."

"One hundred percent oral, love to suck toes, fingers, love to suck and lick ass, swallow cock and his cum."

"I find kissing to be very erotic and like to do it often."

"Kissing is first, I am a great deep-throater."

FANTASIES

"I fantasize about being a sex slave or being so desirable that my sex partner can't help succumbing to me."

"I imagine a guy sucking me off and I cum in his mouth and all over him."

"Simple fantasies usually involving doing vanilla things with a hot muscular partner, sometimes shower scenes, group sex."

WHAT SEX ACTS DO YOU LIKE MOST AND LEAST?

As he is an experimental lover, in addition to his favorite sex acts, oral sex, sixty-nine, and kissing all over the body, he enjoys voyeurism, incorporating costumes and sometimes food. His least favorite sex acts are rough sex and behaviors that involve pain.

"I love mutual masturbation, because you can kiss and

look at each other and see their entire body and think about all the other sex acts, fucking, blowing."

"I like rimming, kissing, and anal sex."

"Kissing first, sucking, fucking, masturbation, face fucking, ball play."

"I don't like biting, pinching, slapping, rough penetration."

AS A LOVER, WHAT'S YOUR BEST SKILL?

What distinguishes Scorpio among other lovers is the way he uses his natural animal magnetism to excite his partner even before any kissing or touching has occurred.

"I have made my partners cum in their pants with just my tongue and hands."

"Teasing, my mouth, kissing, licking, sucking, swallowing, talking dirty."

"I give great massages, all over a guy's body."

"I like to please and be pleased. I am told that I am a very good top due to the curve of my cock."

WHAT SMELLS AND TASTES ON YOUR PARTNER DO YOU ENJOY?

He loves the smell of his partner's skin, his penis, his hair, and certain mild colognes, particularly those with a spicy edge. He also enjoys the taste of natural clean skin.

"I enjoy the smells of his groin and feet as well as the taste of his cum and his skin around the genitals, feet and mouth."

"I love the smell and taste of skin, especially his penis."

"His manly body smells turn me on, sweat, ass, and a good cologne."

"I like the taste of his body juices, sweat, saliva, cum."

A MEMORY

"There was one instance when I chatted with these two men on the Internet. We had discussed meeting for sex. So, after exchanging pictures we agreed to meet. I drove to their house. I walked in and we all chatted for a minute. I then started to blow one of the two men while he was sitting in a chair in the living room. Then the second man came in and I alternated blowing the two of them back and forth. I then went back to blowing the first man. By that time we were all naked. The second guy came up behind me and started to slide his cock into my ass while I continued to blow the first guy. We went like that for some time until I slid out from under the second guy and straddled the first guy who was still sitting in the chair. I rode him for a little bit. At that point we moved to the floor where I got on my back and raised my legs and both men took turns fucking me. Then the first man was ready to cum so he was fucking me and shot his load in my ass. After he finished the second man started to fuck me and blew his load in my ass as well."

FOR SOME PEOPLE THE TASTE OF THEIR PARTNER'S CUM IS UNPLEASANT. IF THAT'S TRUE FOR YOU, WHAT DO YOU DO ABOUT THE TASTE?

Scorpio has no problem with the taste of his partner's cum.

"After shooting on my lips or face, I kiss him with his own cum."

"I swallow if I know the person well or when I'm committed to someone."

"I enjoy the taste of cum and will swallow if I'm in a monogamous relationship."

"I love to taste, swallow my boyfriend's cum."

"I don't find the taste of cum to be unpleasant. I swallow, have it shot or rubbed on me."

"I like the taste of cum, I swallow, rub it on my body or on him."

"I swallow or rub it on myself. Sometimes I jerk off with it."

DO YOU ENJOY WATCHING YOUR PARTNER DURING SEX AND ORGASM? DO YOU ENJOY BEING WATCHED?

This man is visually oriented and has the ability to stare down everyone, everything for that matter, even the family cat. So, of course, he watches his partner closely during the sexual experience. But because of his secretive streak, he doesn't necessarily like to return the favor.

The Big "O"

HOW DO YOU REACH AN ORGASM AND HOW OFTEN?

Scorpio achieves orgasm almost every time he has sex usually through a combination of oral sex and masturbation. For some, anal sex is an integral part of orgasm.

"Pull my balls, I will cum."

WHAT'S YOUR FAVORITE POSITION?

He has no favorite position for orgasm, enjoying spooning, having his partner on top, being on top, or lying side by side. Doggie style is fine too but it may be his least preferred.

SOME PEOPLE ARE CONCERNED ABOUT BRINGING A PARTNER TO CLIMAX BEFORE HAVING AN ORGASM THEMSELVES. OTHERS STRIVE TO REACH ORGASM TOGETHER. WHICH IS TRUE FOR YOU?

Scorpio has considerable control and likes to time it so that he and his partner climax together or almost at the same moment.

"I prefer to reach orgasm together, but often it enhances my pleasure if I help my partner climax first."

"Together, sometimes I like for him to cum first, so I can pay attention to pleasing him 100 percent."

"I don't mind either, as long as the two orgasms are close."

A MEMORY

"I was with a striking, in shape, virile, assertive man who had a huge penis. He rubbed his hands all over my body, fingered my butt hole, and whispered sexual needs and desires. Then gradually he entered my anus with slow penetration."

ARE YOU VOCAL DURING SEX?

True to his secretive nature, Scorpio is not very vocal during sex, mostly making low moans of pleasure.

"I don't say much, but I do groan."

AFTER SEX WHAT DO YOU LIKE TO DO?

He wants to take his time, lounge around for a bit, then go on to other activities.

"I particularly like to nap then get up and head out."

"Afterwards a little talk, shower, take a walk."

"Cuddle, watch TV then a bit later, go out together."

"Go to sleep or do it again after some cuddling and kissing."

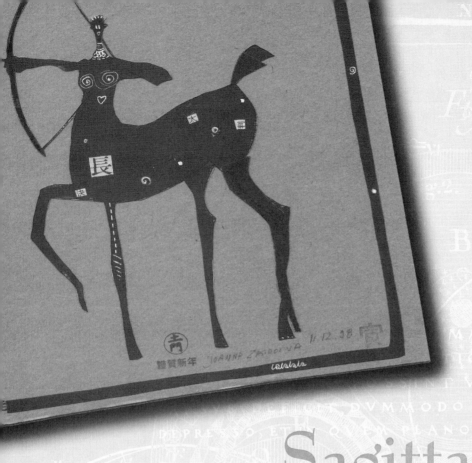

Sagittarius

THE ARCHER

November 22 through December 21

FIRE SIGN SAGITTARIUS is mellow, laid-back, generous, friendly, and forthright. They speak bluntly, without awareness that their words can hurt, striking home like the Archer's arrows. Ruler of the hips and legs in the physical body, Sagittarius loves the outdoors, for hiking, camping, and having sex.

He says: "I am usually complimented on how I kiss. I will kiss or lick any part of a lover's body including the anus. Every part of his body is worthy of love."

"Float like a butterfly.

Sting like a bee."

—Drew "Bundini" Brown,
boxing credo for Muhammad Ali

The Sagittarius Man
in His Own Words

"My partner and I had been together for a long time. On this occasion the encounter lasted for hours before we came. It was late night and we went through periods of hot lovemaking, interspersed with short periods of cuddling and sleeping.

"We explored each other's bodies over and over again, kissing, cuddling, performing oral sex, mutual and solo stroking, and deep mutual rimming, with him straddling me. The hottest part was how we shared breath. We faced each other as if kissing. When he exhaled, I inhaled and vice-versa. We weren't totally lip-locked when doing this, some mix of air came in. This was a heady, erotic experience.

"While sharing breath, we were also gently feeling each other up. Then after about five hours, and wonderful release, I was in a relaxed and blissful state for the rest of the day. I loved the smell of every bit of his body and I loved the scent of his cum on my stomach and chest."

Attraction and Dating a Sagittarius

WHAT ATTRACTS YOU TO SOMEONE?

Sagittarius is an outgoing Fire Sign and all Fire Signs are quite physical. As a result, a man's health and looks are important to him. He sums up his list of attractive features under the heading of "a nice body," but what he notices most is the muscles of the legs.

"He should possess all his teeth and hair, be self-assured and a good conversationalist, and have an outgoing personality, mature. I prefer a man who is in decent shape. I'm not into bear types."

"A well-built, good-looking man with an average penis size pleases me. Briefs are a big turn-on."

"I like men who are taller than I am and bigger, but not fat. I'm indifferent to hair; I like both hairy and smooth. Well-developed bodies also turn me on."

"Musculature. I like men who know what they want, who are sensitive, caring and loving, who will take charge at times, but are also willing to follow."

"I am attracted to a good-looking man who has a nice body. His penis size really doesn't matter unless it is minute."

"Brown eyes, naturally toned bodies, brown hair, tattoos, good-sized penis, high sexual energy, at times submissive, at times aggressive, respectful behavior."

WHAT MIGHT TURN YOU OFF?

Since Sagittarius is a relaxed man, outgoing but not aggressive, men who are pushy, arrogant, or clingy really turn him off. The Archer also has a broad spectrum of interests, which might include politics, travel, and gambling. A man who is home-centered or a couch potato will bore Sagittarius.

"I dislike people who have low self-esteem and express it as meanness or by being distrustful and suspicious."

"Lack of class, lack of common courtesy and dishonesty all turn me off."

"Skinny, milquetoast, effeminate."

"Overweight, unclean, wimpy, laziness, self-pity, users."

"Smoking turns me off, dirty appearance and extreme overweight, although a sweet, gentle, overweight guy is okay."

WHAT DO YOU ENJOY DOING ON A DATE?

He has wide-ranging interests, which usually include travel. This is a man who loves to decide at 9 a.m. on a Saturday to pack a bag and head out of town for the weekend. Therefore, spontaneity is an important part of any evening out and sex is an important part of the night.

"Going out to eat, having sex if there is a strong attraction."

"Dining out, walking, good conversation, cuddling, hugging, and sex."

"Sex, sex, sex, sex, etc.—sex."

"Food, films, quiet get-togethers with a small number of good friends."

"Getting to know the person for who he is, talking, going on long walks."

"Going to the movies, out to dinner, going out almost anywhere, staying home watching TV."

ARE YOU FLIRTATIOUS?

Sagittarius is by nature laid-back and mellow. When it comes to flirtation, his behavior is seldom over the top, but he is mildly so.

"I can be, to an extent. I like to make people laugh."

"I am flirtatious sometimes, but not too much."

ARE YOU JEALOUS?

In spite of his quiet self-assured demeanor, this man has a jealous streak. It almost comes as a surprise to him when these feelings surface because his nature is generally so laid-back. The point is that Sagittarius is fundamentally trusting. He isn't going to do something behind his partner's back so he doesn't expect his partner to betray him.

"Yes, to a certain extent. You can look, but don't touch."

"Yes, somewhat. In a serious, long-term relationship where there is a commitment, I could see myself feeling possessive."

HOW DO YOU FEEL ABOUT PUBLIC DISPLAYS OF AFFECTION?

Stay home if you want to get physical. This is not pleasing to him as a participant or an observer.

"Some things are better left at home."

"If it's a minor kiss or hug I don't mind. If it is very deep or sexual I think they should get a room."

"I shy away from them and generally don't view them as appropriate."

"I won't display affection publicly. Being part of a gay couple, I am unwilling to invite controversy."

"I'm not interested. It makes me uncomfortable."

Sexual Attitudes and Behaviors

HOW OFTEN DO YOU THINK ABOUT SEX AND HOW OFTEN PER WEEK DO YOU WANT TO HAVE SEX?

He thinks about sex frequently in the course of a day and would love to have it daily, but given time constraints he usually settles for three or four sessions weekly.

A MEMORY

"One of my most memorable encounters was with a guy who loves to have his ass eaten out. I used my big tongue to satisfy him. He had a most suckable ass. We went on like that for what seemed like hours. Later on, I fucked him and delighted at watching my cock slide in an out of his sweet white ass."

HOW MUCH TIME DO YOU LIKE TO SPEND HAVING SEX AND HOW MUCH OF THAT TIME IS FOREPLAY? DO YOU ENJOY QUICKIES?

Optimum time for sex is thirty to forty minutes with about fifteen to twenty-five minutes spent on foreplay. He never objects to quickies and on occasion enjoys longer sex sessions, lasting perhaps two hours.

"Quickies are fine with me. I like sex as often as I can get it. I like to mix foreplay and sex the entire time."

"Quick or long, I like all of it. Foreplay varies in length of time."

"How much time I spend varies, it depends on our mood. I like cuddling sessions and lots of foreplay with the right person."

"I'd say one to one and a half hours total for sex with just fifteen minutes to a half hour of foreplay and, yes quickies are fine."

"I like to spend hours having sex with twenty to thirty minutes minimum for foreplay."

WHAT TIME OF DAY DO YOU PREFER TO HAVE SEX?

He has no preference as to the time for sex. All that matters is not being hurried. Even when having a quickie, the rush is more about urgency than lack of adequate time.

"Nighttime mostly, but I enjoy it during the day too."

"Late afternoon, into evening, but any time will do."

"During the day, especially on the weekend."

"What time is it?"

HOW OFTEN PER WEEK DO YOU MASTURBATE?

When he has a partner, he seldom masturbates. When he is single his average is four times a week.

HOW LONG DO YOU WANT TO KNOW SOMEONE BEFORE GETTING SEXUAL?

In keeping with the impulsive aspect of a Fire Sign and the fact that Sagittarius is a bit of a gambler, he is likely to become sexual with a new partner in very little time, probably on a first date.

"Not long at all, one date."

"Are you available?"

"There is no set time that I put on knowing someone before becoming sexual. With some people I had sex right away. There were others I knew for a long time first."

"It usually happens on first contact."

"Within the first week."

WHAT'S YOUR ATTITUDE TOWARD CASUAL SEX?

As it stands to reason for a man who enters sexual relationships in short order and who is apt to go through a promiscuous period, he enjoys casual sex.

A MEMORY

"I met a man at the Vault one night. Like me, he was into leather. He was older, confident, not afraid to go after what he wanted, but also open and friendly. He invited me back to his place, stating that he could be a gentle lover. I took him up on his offer and we had a fun time—oral sex and jerking him off. Then we cuddled and talked for hours. He really listened and seemed to understand me. I spent the night. We horsed around, shared a tub in the morning, and talked some more. He was a nice guy."

"If people are safe, I think it is fine."

"It is fine, although I would like to eventually settle down."

"As long as it is safe it is okay."

"I am single. It is fine."

A FANTASY

"I imagine a guy who is mature, in good shape, and open to expressing himself. I get turned on by that kind of man when he describes his fantasies. Over the last year I have been flirting with a cowboy via the Internet. We talk about him riding into town wearing just his chaps and hat and paying a visit to me at the local watering hole. My fantasies consist of silly fun stuff like that."

DO YOU BELIEVE IN MONOGAMY?

Known as the bachelor Sign of the zodiac, whose symbol is the centaur, Sagittarius is in no hurry to settle down. Once committed, however, he strives to be loyal to his partner.

"Yes I do, although I know it can be hard to find someone who wants to settle down."

"I believe that monogamy is a couple's choice and that having many lovers is equally valid."

"Yes and no, because, some sex outside a relationship can make sex with your partner more exciting."

"Yes, for one thing you don't have to worry about protecting yourself."

"Yes, with the right person. It must be mutual with both of us believing 'I live for thee and thee alone.'"

DOES SEX HAVE A SPIRITUAL SIGNIFICANCE FOR YOU?

Sagittarius loves casual sex, which is exciting and often fulfilling but purely physical. When he is single, therefore, he does not see a spiritual aspect to sex. When in a committed and loving relationship, his attitude changes.

"With the right person I do enjoy a deeper bond."

"Yes, I can feel my heart opening as I think about this question. I believe that our life purpose is to learn to give and receive love. Sex is one way to share love."

"Yes, it does, when two are united in a sexual act, it involves all of humanness, including their spiritual being."

"Yes, there is a kind of connection that is transcending during climax."

ARE YOU COMFORTABLE INITIATING SEXUAL ACTIVITIES?

His nature is easy going and his interactions in a newly forming relationship are seldom aggressive and yet, in most situations, he is quite comfortable initiating sex.

HOW DO YOU COMMUNICATE TO YOUR PARTNER YOUR SEXUAL WANTS AND NEEDS?

He tends to be receptive to his partner during sex and is therefore more likely to communicate with gestures than with words to make his desires known.

"I do to my partner what I like done to me. It usually works."

"I usually let him do what he wants."

DO YOU THINK OF YOURSELF AS BEING IN THE MAINSTREAM SEXUALLY, MORE EXPERIMENTAL, OPEN TO ANYTHING?

He is an experimental lover open to anal sex both as top and bottom. He enjoys participating in a ménage à trois, being with a hairy man and is into interracial sex. In addition he is turned on by sex in public places such as doing it in the woods or on the beach. When it comes to sex toys, his collection is usually limited to dildoes and vibrators.

In his fantasy life, he imagines anonymous sex and scenes of dominance and submission.

> ### FANTASIES
>
> "My fantasy is to get fucked and be blown and blow someone else all at the same time."
>
> "I have always had a fantasy about being stopped by a cop. Then he and I get it on in the woods."
>
> "I imagine having sex outside, for example, on a mountain path or while drifting in a boat on the river."
>
> "Being dominated by a hot, sexy aggressive man and then dominating him in turn."

HOW DO YOU DEMONSTRATE AFFECTION FOR YOUR PARTNER?

With Sagittarius, actions speak louder than words. He demonstrates affection in ways that indicate his awareness of his partner's wants and needs. He might touch his lover tenderly or offer a massage, cook him a meal, or buy him a small gift.

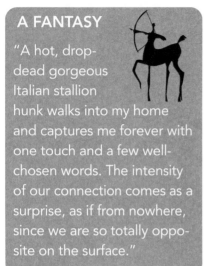

A FANTASY

"A hot, drop-dead gorgeous Italian stallion hunk walks into my home and captures me forever with one touch and a few well-chosen words. The intensity of our connection comes as a surprise, as if from nowhere, since we are so totally opposite on the surface."

"By doing unexpected things, visiting at will, bringing him dinner or buying something for him unexpectedly."

"Some physical act each day and, when possible or appropriate, kisses, hugs, back massage throughout the day. I cook things that I know he will enjoy. To me that is also an expression of affection."

"Kissing, hugging, finding out what my partner is feeling, stroking my partner's body, giving a neck rub."

"Gifts of food, gifts of consciousness, gifts of positive intentions, gifts of beauty."

The Five Senses

HOW IMPORTANT TO YOU IS THE SEXUAL ENVIRONMENT?

Most of the time Sagittarius prefers that the sexual environment be clean and comfortable. He is, however, a bit of a gambler and there are times when, in the heat of the moment, lust will overtake any reservations.

"For casual sex I am less picky. For romantic encounters I like my privacy and safety."

"Very important, clean, somewhat orderly, doesn't have to be ornate or fancy."

"Lighting is important. I like to have sex in a dimly lighted setting not in absolute darkness. Having sex in the dark feels weird to me."

"The place must be clean."

WHERE DO YOU LIKE TO HAVE SEX?

In general, Sagittarius prefers his creature comforts and chooses to have sex in the comfort of a bedroom. For quickies or casual sex, anywhere will do.

"Any place that is warm and comfortable."

"Bed is best. I've done it outdoors. That's exciting but risky. I like it least of all in cars."

"In the shower, swimming pools, or a Jacuzzi."

"Most often in bed, but almost anywhere is okay."

WHAT PUTS YOU IN THE MOOD FOR SEX?

The fundamental nature of Sagittarius is easy going but also highly sexual. He would be happy to have sex daily, so when he is in the company of someone he finds attractive and he feels relaxed, he is in the mood.

"Taking a shower together, watching porn videos, and foreplay."

"I am a very sexual person. I don't need things to arouse me, just a touch will do."

"Quiet, pleasant place, moderately low light, showering, porn, low levels of any pleasant scent."

"It just kind of falls into place and it has to feel good and upbeat, having plenty of time. Desire is pretty much always there. The opportunity to act on it is not."

> ## A FANTASY
>
> "My fantasies are different all the time. They frequently involve famous athletes, such as baseball or hockey players. A recent one featured two very well known heterosexual baseball Hall of Famers. One man is fucking the other up the ass. After he climaxes I have the pleasure to suck out the cum."

"Almost anything, but mostly being close to someone I find attractive."

"Showers, candles, food, especially seafood. Porn is a stimulant but I don't need it to put me in the mood."

"I am always in the mood for sex."

WHAT'S YOUR ATTITUDE TOWARD PORNOGRAPHY?

He enjoys pornography, especially when masturbating. The imagery that turns him on most is of dominate muscular men, bikers, or police officers, in out-of-the-ordinary settings, such as beside a stream or across the hood of a car.

"It can be fun every now and then."

"At times I have loved it, at times not. Now that I am in a relationship I don't have much interest in it. When I was single I used it quite a lot."

"I like it. Sometimes porn is my only outlet."

HOW MUCH CUDDLING DO YOU ENJOY, ASIDE FROM SEX?

Sagittarius is the don't-fence-me-in Sign of the zodiac. Although it is important to him to share affection with a lover, a hug, holding hands, and cuddling, a little goes a long way.

"I want a little each day, even if it is just a long hug or squeeze."

HOW TACTILE AND HOW ORAL ARE YOU?

Sagittarius may derive a bit more pleasure from the experience of touching his lover's body with his hands rather than with his mouth, but when it comes to oral sex he excels.

"Oh, yes, yes, yes. I am very tactile. I am very much into body contact and affection. I am also very oral. I love deep kissing, kissing my partner's body all over, even armpits, if he is really clean. I am only into rimming if I have gotten to know the guy and feel safe."

"I am very tactile. Whether a man's skin is smooth or hairy, they are both erotic to me. I enjoy all things oral. I will lick any part of a lover's body, including the anus. Every part of his body is worthy of love."

"I am both very tactile and very oral. I like to taste my partner."

"I am very tactile and love running my hands over his body. It turns me on too when he reciprocates. I also enjoy all aspects of oral sex from kissing to rimming."

WHAT SEX ACTS DO YOU LIKE MOST AND LEAST?

What's not to like about sex? He's a very open lover. About the only thing that doesn't interest him is using sex toys.

"Kissing, oral sex, mutual masturbation, fondling. Any type of body contact, '69,' rubbing penises together, cuddling."

"I would say in order of preference, kissing, oral sex, mutual masturbation, and anal sex."

"So far, there isn't anything I don't like about sex."

AS A LOVER, WHAT'S YOUR BEST SKILL?

One of his skills is his spontaneity, his responsiveness to the opportunity for sex at any time of day and in almost any location. Beyond that, he is a good lover in virtually all aspects.

"My skill is being in tune with partner, knowing what feels right to him so that he is comfortable and can enjoy it more."

"I focus on my partner's pleasure and invariably that increases mine. I love to use my hands and mouth all over his body."

"My mouth, whether I am biting slightly, licking, or giving passionate kisses."

"I am a good sucker."

WHAT SMELLS AND TASTES ON YOUR PARTNER DO YOU ENJOY?

He enjoys the smell of his partner's skin and the scent of his lover on his clothes. Most often he prefers the simple aroma of his lover's skin without colognes. When it comes to tastes, again his preference is unadorned body tastes and he rarely chooses to incorporate food into his sex play.

"I love the smell of a clean man's crotch. The anus can be pleasant, depending on the guy. Any natural scent on a clean man, even the armpits, is great. I love the taste of my partner's mouth, his body in general and crotch. The taste and feel of pre-cum can be very stimulating and exciting."

"I like the smell of colognes and sometimes the smell of an unwashed, uncut cock and the musky smell around the testicles. I like the taste of his cum and his underarms."

FANTASIES

"I have several, all focus around a big, bulky man. Meeting such a man naked, while hiking or canoeing in a forested area. Meeting such a man in leather, on a motorcycle, or having such a man appearing at my door in short shorts only and taking me."

"I am being brought to climax by a doctor during a routine medical examination. Sometimes I fantasize about having a three-way with a woman and another man. In yet another fantasy, I am watching nude wrestling or nude diving, or Olympic games as they were performed in ancient Greece."

"The smell of his skin, that musky scent from the genital area, is very appealing to me and I like the tastes over all his body."

"I don't like baby powder or deodorant to interfere with natural smells. I like some colognes, woodsy, spicy. I also like the smells on his clothes around the penis area."

FOR SOME PEOPLE THE TASTE OF THEIR PARTNER'S CUM IS UNPLEASANT. IF THAT'S TRUE FOR YOU, WHAT DO YOU DO ABOUT THE TASTE?

He rarely has any difficulty with the taste of cum, and when he is with a partner that he knows well, he swallows.

"It doesn't bother me at all. If it does, I just grab a towel. I love to play with cum and I swallow."

"I don't mind the taste of cum. I love cumming into my partner's body and love having his cum anywhere on my body."

"Taste is no problem for me. I swallow cum or rub it on my own penis to use it as a lubricant for masturbation. It is a great lubricant."

"I find taste depends upon the food my partner has eaten. Pineapple sweetens his cum. I rub it on myself and swallow it."

FANTASIES

"I get really excited thinking about cumming into my partner in any way and having him cum into me. Thoughts of water sports are also very erotic. Whenever I see a hot guy, I imagine smelling his crotch. What a turn-on!"

"One fantasy I have is being with a bodybuilder, someone anonymous, and slowly stripping him."

DO YOU ENJOY WATCHING YOUR PARTNER DURING SEX AND ORGASM? DO YOU ENJOY BEING WATCHED?

As a man who enjoys a range of sexual experiences that are experimental, including having sex in public places and ménage à trois, he definitely wants to observe his partner during sex and orgasm. Being watched in return is okay but a bit less comfortable.

The Big "O"
· ·

HOW DO YOU REACH AN ORGASM AND HOW OFTEN?

Oral sex will do it, so will anal sex, and masturbation always works as well.

"I almost always reach orgasm whether by oral sex, self- or mutual masturbation, or by rubbing my penis on my partner's body."

WHAT IS YOUR FAVORITE POSITION?

In addition to "69," which is his favorite, he enjoys spooning, stomach to back, and doggie style.

SOME PEOPLE ARE VERY CONCERNED ABOUT BRINGING THEIR PARTNER TO CLIMAX BEFORE HAVING AN ORGASM THEMSELVES. OTHERS STRIVE TO REACH ORGASM TOGETHER. WHICH IS TRUE FOR YOU?

Sagittarius is far too easygoing to be concerned about who cums first. He is attentive to his lover, cares that he reach climax and fully expects to have an orgasm as well, but first, last, or together doesn't matter.

"As long as everyone gets pleasured, I am very happy with that."

"It is different all the time. I am okay if it doesn't happen simultaneously."

"Ideally reaching orgasm together, but definitely I prefer to get my partner off first."

ARE YOU VOCAL DURING SEX?

Sagittarius isn't shy about asking for what he wants, but when it comes to expressing pleasure, his lover will know more from his behavior than from words that he is content.

"I am vocal, but not verbal. I like to express pleasure with grunting and groaning. I will speak a little to ask about my partner's pleasure or to ask for something."

AFTER SEX WHAT DO YOU LIKE TO DO?

He prefers unhurried activities before going to sleep. With a new partner, he appreciates a man who will stay with him for a while before going home.

"I love to stay with him, cuddle, sleep, anything. But typically guys just want to leave after they finish up."

"It's nice to cuddle, listen to music, talk softly, give a massage, perhaps take a hot shower then go to sleep."

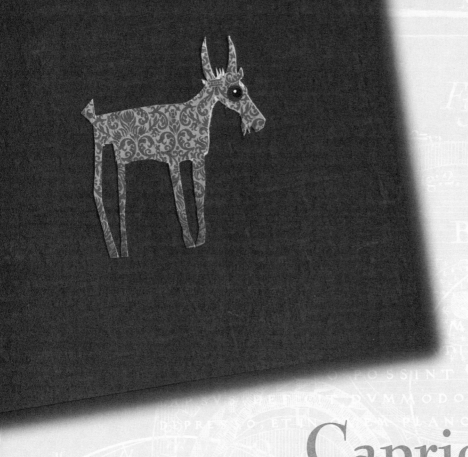

Capricorn

THE GOAT

December 22 through January 19

EARTH SIGN CAPRICORN, thoughtful, practical, ambitious, has great integrity. Ruler of the knees in particular and the whole skeletal system, Capricorn loves exploring all of the body with his hands and tongue. The hardest workers in the zodiac, they put effort into everything they do, including being great lovers.

What he says: "I love passion, laying together, feeling him on top of me, making out, a bit of rough sex thrown in."

"Sex is like money; only too much is enough."

—John Updike

The Capricorn Man
in His Own Words

A MEMORY

"The sexual encounter that most sticks out in my mind took place in a sauna in Amsterdam. I was with a striking blond muscle boy. We took a shower together and soaped up each other's body. We then started rubbing up against one another, his hard cock against mine was so exciting. We continued like that, deep kissing as well, until we both came. What heightened the whole experience was the fact that we were being watched by other men who were jacking off. It was a hot scene."

Attraction and Dating a Capricorn

● ●

WHAT ATTRACTS YOU TO SOMEONE?

Capricorn cares about what other people think. He is, therefore, attracted to a man who is careful about his appearance, who presents himself appropriately in public. What turns his head is a strong-looking man, a man he describes as masculine, perhaps defined by muscles and a good physique.

"It is the whole package—a guy's butt, his hands, eyes, big ears, lips, thick necks. I like pronounced Adam's apples, stubble, big forearms, and beyond the physical, a passion for life, and an open mind."

"Athleticism, muscles, a kind-looking face and a great smile. Big arms that I can feel safe in are a major plus."

"I am attracted to a man with a well-defined physique, clear eyes, strong voice, smile, a confident inner self."

"Masculine men with dark hair and eyes, height in proportion to weight, easygoing, a sense of humor, energetic, and affectionate."

"Dark hair, youthful look, eyes, smile, manly voice. I like masculine men."

"Personality, sense of humor, hairy chest, taller than me, rugged build."

MEMORIES

"We were making love in a lightning storm. All my senses seemed heightened and I remember the smell of sweet grass, the feel and the aroma of fragrant breezes, the sound of rustling leaves, the breathing rhythm of my lover, and an all over wonderful sense of calm."

"What comes to mind was a long slow foreplay session, including mutual actions, male breasts and nipples, slow and satisfying '69' and then fucking each other in turn."

"We have been married for eighteen years and the sex is always good. Sometimes we simply have raw sex where we just want to be inside the other person's body."

WHAT MIGHT TURN YOU OFF?

On the surface, Capricorn may appear somewhat conservative, quiet, perhaps reserved. Underneath it all he has considerable ambition and a strong sex drive. A man who lacks direction won't hold his attention.

"Loud people or bossy people put me off as do men who are overweight, self centered, or selfish."

"What turns me off most of all is poor attention to teeth, that and fem behavior."

"Someone who is not clean, feminine guys."

"Arrogant gay men with attitude and not being friendly."

"Physically dirty and bad breath, smoking. I want nothing to do with a man who is drunk or high."

"Overweight or very skinny, bad teeth."

WHAT DO YOU ENJOY DOING ON A DATE?

Capricorn likes the finer things, good food, a pleasant environment for dinner, a nice bottle of wine. In fact in a long-term relationship, he would love to take a cruise, visit neighboring mansions, or spend time at a resort on a secluded beach. Whether in a new relationship or a long-term one, he especially enjoys spending quiet time with his lover.

"I enjoy going on a hike, having dinner by candlelight, sitting in a café, holding hands, a bit of serious conversation, and staring into someone's eyes."

"Conversation, strolling in the park or garden, taking in a movie, having a picnic on the beach, going cycling, or taking a boat cruise."

"Movies, long walks together, romantic dinners, going to the beach, and staying the night there."

"Eating dinner, wine, dancing, walking, sight seeing, nature related (beach, woods) museums."

"Talking over dinner, going for a walk, only kissing on the first date."

"Dinner, talk, sharing, and then on to sex."

ARE YOU FLIRTATIOUS?

He is somewhat flirtatious, but he is, by nature, a quiet man and his overtures are rather subtle.

"Yes, I am flirtatious but moderately so and, perhaps this seems strange, but I am least flirtatious around the people I am attracted to because I choke up."

"Sometimes I am. I love to flirt with my eyes and by touching someone in a certain way."

"Yes, but not that much. I would say that I can be flirtatious if the situation calls for it."

"I think that I am, casually so, with good friends."

ARE YOU JEALOUS?

Capricorn comes across as inherently self-confident, but there is a seldom seen yet deep-seated core of insecurity in his nature, and he can be somewhat jealous. It is not usually a major issue, nonetheless, he will admit that jealousy is a bit of a problem for him.

"Sometimes I can be very jealous. Yes."

"Yes, but I am trying not to be."

HOW DO YOU FEEL ABOUT PUBLIC DISPLAYS OF AFFECTION?

The Goat is a very private individual and concerned about proper behavior, so overt displays must stay within limits. He is also practical and, for the sake of safety, is guarded in public.

A FANTASY

"I would like to fulfill this fantasy—to have a threesome with two men double penetrating me in my ass with their cocks and cumming in me. I imagine making love with both of them all night long, in bed, and putting our tongues in each other's mouths. I picture my lover and me sucking the third man's cock, or me sucking his balls while my partner sucks his cock. Maybe someday . . ."

"In my opinion, hand holding and flirting is great. Kissing heavily or more is rude."

"I would love to show my affection in public, but it is not accepted anywhere. I think that's, unfortunate."

"I feel uncomfortable about openly showing my affection for another man. I fear being attacked."

"They are fine within limits, specifically in a gay-friendly environment."

Sexual Attitudes and Behaviors

FANTASIES

"My fantasies include being with a straight man who licks my ass then fucks it for hours after he has just had sex with a woman."

"I imagine someone realizing that he has been in love with me all his life, who then makes passionate love to me while tears of joy are flowing down his cheeks."

"Teasing a man so much that he cums without my even having touched him."

HOW OFTEN DO YOU THINK ABOUT SEX AND HOW OFTEN PER WEEK DO YOU WANT SEX?

Capricorn is quite sexual by nature. He has sex on the brain daily and he'd enjoy having sex every day. If time precludes that, he'll settle for five times per week.

"I want it seven times . . . actually, whenever available."

HOW LONG DO YOU LIKE TO SPEND HAVING SEX AND HOW MUCH OF THAT TIME IS FOREPLAY? DO YOU ENJOY QUICKIES?

Quickies are not his favorite, as he prefers sex that lasts a minimum of one half hour. He loves occasional marathons as well. Foreplay ranges from short to long depending on the circumstances.

"I prefer taking my time, enjoying the experience. Quickies are good every once in a while."

"A half hour is best but I enjoy quickies if nothing else is available."

"I love spending a long time, an hour or two."

"Hours, if we have all night, sometimes just five to ten minutes can be fun."

WHAT TIME OF DAY DO YOU PREFER TO HAVE SEX?

As he doesn't like to be rushed when having sex; he prefers encounters when his mind isn't on having to be somewhere else; before he becomes overly tired, such as mornings and evenings.

"My favorite times for sex are at night and when I just wake up."

"I prefer between six and nine in the morning, between nine and eleven at night."

"First thing in the morning or in the evening just before falling asleep."

HOW OFTEN PER WEEK DO YOU MASTURBATE?

He masturbates on average four times per week with periods when he does it daily and others when he does it rarely.

HOW LONG DO YOU WANT TO KNOW SOMEONE BEFORE GETTING SEXUAL?

By nature Capricorn is cautious but he also trusts his gut feelings, so this decision is made based upon how soon he feels comfortable with a man. That is not likely to be on a first date, but two dates is generally enough for him to know whether sex is appealing with a new man.

"It depends. I have done it after just meeting someone and I have waited until several weeks of dating."

"I would say from a few hours up to one month, depending."

"The norm for me is two dates, but then again it really depends on the level of attraction I am feeling for a man."

MEMORIES

"We were in a cabin near the beach. It was right around sundown and there was a cool breeze coming through the window and the open door. We lit candles, and my partner and I took our time, talking, kissing, touching, getting more intense as time passed."

"Piggy sex, words mixed with water sports, bareback, dildoes."

"We had gone camping, hiked for a while, and then went swimming. When we came back to our site, we had sex on the picnic table. His body had a salty flavor from the beach. It was a bit risky because it was daylight, and there were people nearby."

WHAT'S YOUR ATTITUDE TOWARD CASUAL SEX?

He doesn't deny that it's risky but he has a very strong sex drive and, therefore, engages in anonymous sex. Images of casual sex frequently fill his fantasies.

"I love it as long as it is done safely."

"It's great, but I don't do it anymore. Too unsafe."

DO YOU BELIEVE IN MONOGAMY?

The intimacy, comfort, security, and richness that can be found in a monogamous relationship are of real value to him. He finds it hard to achieve such a partnership. He has a practical attitude about monogamy, however. It is not a "make it or break it" part of a relationship.

"Yes. Monogamy is great if you can get it. It is an ideal."

"If two people are sexually and spiritually compatible, monogamy is the way to go."

"I do, for the most part, but if someone slips up once in a while, it would not be the end of the world."

"Yes, I do. Monogamy is great. It is both fulfilling and safe."

DOES SEX HAVE A SPIRITUAL SIGNIFICANCE FOR YOU?

This is a man who keeps his feelings in check and is slow to reveal them. He is pragmatic and may seem dry, but when someone touches his heart, a surprisingly warm and loving nature is revealed. Sex has a definitely spiritual aspect.

"Yes, because both sex and spirituality are about love and connection, a way of extending outside oneself."

"Sometimes. With the right person and if we touch our souls when having sex, then yes it feels spiritual."

"It is God's greatest gift."

"Yes, because sex is nurturing and it unites the souls."

"This depends on who I am with. If it is someone I care for, yes, it does have a spiritual significance."

"I believe that when you love someone, receiving and giving pleasure brings you closer to God."

ARE YOU COMFORTABLE INITIATING SEXUAL ACTIVITIES?

Capricorn has a way of sizing up a situation without anyone knowing that he is doing it. Proverbially, he keeps his cards close to his chest. This is true when it comes to deciding whether to approach a man for sex. He watches body language cues and listens attentively. Then, trusting his instincts, feeling that he won't be rejected, he is comfortable initiating.

HOW DO YOU COMMUNICATE TO YOUR PARTNER YOUR SEXUAL WANTS AND NEEDS?

When it comes to communicating about sex, here too Capricorn uses his instincts to figure out what his partner wants. With considerable subtlety, he uses gestures more than words to indicate what's working for him.

"I use some of both, but I must admit, I do not do enough of either."

DO YOU THINK OF YOURSELF AS BEING IN THE MAINSTREAM SEXUALLY, MORE EXPERIMENTAL, OR OPEN TO ANYTHING?

He is quite experimental in his range of sexuality. He will use vibrators and dildoes, and both give and receive anal sex. Costumes such as underwear and leather and latex may be part of his sex play. He is turned on by hairy men and will try a ménage à trois, perhaps an orgy. In the right settings he is willing to have sex in public places, participate in exhibitionism, try a bit of bondage, dominance, and submission.

His fantasy world usually incorporates some degree of aggression, from mild scenes of master and slave interaction all the way to sadomasochism.

FANTASIES

"My fantasies involve passion, lying together, feeling him on top of me, making out, and with a bit of rough sex thrown in."

"I imagine a situation in which I take charge. I like being called 'Sir.'"

"They are about me being tied down, forced to do various things, or being raped."

"Scenes that turn me on incorporate leather, cigars, fisting, toys, and water sports."

"S & M, cock and ball torture, fisting."

HOW DO YOU DEMONSTRATE AFFECTION FOR YOUR PARTNER?

Capricorn shows his caring by helping his partner, quietly participating, without waiting to be asked and without drawing attention to himself. He might clean the house, prepare supper, or show his respect for his partner's need for privacy and simply stay out of the way.

"Making dinner, attentive listening, verbal playfulness and banter, and pet names."

"I clean up after him, touch, loving words, cards, flowers, phone calls, constant communication."

"I am attentive. I get things for him and help out, however he needs. I am there for him and I buy little tokens to remind him how much I care."

"Small gifts, giving him a massage without being asked."

"I try to maintain the house the way he likes it, and I give him space."

"By doing special things for him, making him feel appreciated and wanted."

"I do things for him that he does not like to do, such as his laundry."

The Five Senses

HOW IMPORTANT TO YOU IS THE SEXUAL ENVIRONMENT?

Things like romantic settings including dim lights, incense, and soft music, while they may be appreciated, are by no means necessary for Capricorn. He does appreciate privacy and cleanliness.

"The importance of the setting depends on my mood, but if I had to choose one important factor, it would be cleanliness."

"Clean and private are important. That's about all."

"As long as it is not a garbage dump I won't complain."

"I love clean places, happy colors, and romantic music."

"Cleanliness is of utmost importance, safety too."

WHERE DO YOU LIKE TO HAVE SEX?

Number 1: the bedroom. The traditional Capricorn may be willing to have sex beyond those four walls but he certainly is not the man who wants to do it in glass elevators or any really out of the ordinary place. He wants privacy, comfort, and safety so he can enjoy slow, steady, and fulfilling sessions. The Goat who is more experimental in his sexual nature will enjoy exhibitionism in sex clubs or other safe settings.

"Anywhere in the house is great, also hotels."

"I like to vary the place a little, bathroom, living room."

"Bed most often, but also outdoors such as on the beach or in the woods, in cars and motels."

A MEMORY

"I met a very big muscular guy in a porn shop. We went into a booth and without saying a word, he made it clear that I was to service him all over. He had just come from a gym and had that natural sweaty body smell that I love. I worked his whole body with my mouth. Then he turned me around and fucked my ass very roughly. It was great."

WHAT PUTS YOU IN THE MOOD FOR SEX?

Capricorn thinks about sex every day and doesn't often enjoy quickies. So putting him in the mood for sex requires little other than having adequate time. Pornography, perhaps playing quietly in the background, heightens his mood.

"Porn is good when I masturbate. Sharing food, candlelight, and music are great to set me up for lovemaking."

"Spending time with someone I care about, having dinner, maybe dancing, porn too."

"All that is necessary is being in a warm relaxed place and having time available."

"You name it, it puts me in the mood. I'm always ready."

"The place may put me in the mood but most often it's an aroma; I love good sweaty crotch or under foreskin smells."

"Thinking of my man and just looking at him is all it takes."

"Watching porn videos, music, being relaxed with a glass of wine, a massage."

WHAT'S YOUR ATTITUDE TOWARD PORNOGRAPHY?

His response to pornography ranges from moderate to great interest, but he isn't likely to use it when he is with a partner.

"I have some interest. It can relieve horniness. I would not say that it's a big part of my life."

"Pornography is fine. In fact I love it."

HOW MUCH CUDDLING DO YOU ENJOY, ASIDE FROM SEX?

He loves to touch and be touched, giving little touches as he passes by his lover. He also likes hugs and embraces and lying together at night, even without sexual contact.

"I love to cuddle all the time."

"A lot; touch is more important than orgasm."

"I'll take as much as I can get."

HOW TACTILE AND HOW ORAL ARE YOU?

Capricorn is an Earth Sign and is known for his earthy approach to sex. He pretty much wants to touch, smell, and taste it all.

"I'm extremely tactile and quite oral. I love kissing all over my lover's body as well as deep kissing on the mouth and fellatio."

"I find touch very arousing and I am very oral. For me kissing comes first, blow jobs second, and rimming third."

"I am very oral and love French kissing, licking, and oral sex. I'm not too much into rimming."

WHAT SEX ACTS DO YOU LIKE MOST AND LEAST?

He likes most everything about sex, and for many Capricorns that includes going beyond vanilla sex into a range of fetishes. It is, however, the minority of Capricorns who are into the most open of sexual activities, those involving sado-masochism, water sports, or fisting.

"I love kissing and full body contact, pretty much everything except fondling breasts."

"Kissing is great, so are oral sex and mutual masturbation. Anal sex comes second and nipple play last."

"I'm not into fisting and pain, golden showers, or S&M stuff."

"I don't like any act that involves the mouth in contact with the anus."

AS A LOVER, WHAT'S YOUR BEST SKILL?

Capricorn doesn't rush. He lingers lovingly over his kisses and foreplay, all the way to carefully controlled oral and anal sex.

"I give the best blow jobs."

"Kissing and oral sex are my best. I have also been told I'm really good at being the top or bottom."

"Great at anal sex."

"My mouth, oral, kissing, and rimming."

"Cock sucking, receptive anal."

WHAT SMELLS AND TASTES ON YOUR PARTNER DO YOU ENJOY?

He is very physical. He loves the smells and tastes of his partner's body as he gets more and more excited. Colognes and after-shave aren't likely to turn him on.

"The smell of skin, hair, crotch, clean cock and balls, and his underwear all excite me."

"The smell of his underarms, his hair and crotch area, the taste of his natural juices and sweat."

"Skin, crotch, testicles, and penis under a ripe foreskin."

"I love the smell of his skin, especially in the groin area, neck, chest, arms."

"Taste of butt and foreskin."

FOR SOME PEOPLE THE TASTE OF THEIR PARTNER'S CUM IS UNPLEASANT. IF THAT'S TRUE FOR YOU, WHAT DO YOU DO ABOUT THE TASTE?

Capricorn is earthy by disposition and most often he has no trouble with the taste of cum. He may choose to avoid taking it in his mouth for safety reasons.

"I like my partner's cum and swallow or rub it on him or on me."

"I like it and use it to masturbate."

"Used to always swallow, now for health reasons, I rub it on him."

"I love to swallow, masturbate with it, rub it all over."

"Sometimes I swallow or let it drip out of my mouth and show it to my partner."

"I do not prefer the taste and rarely swallow. I may rub it on myself, depending on the person I'm with."

DO YOU ENJOY WATCHING YOUR PARTNER DURING SEX AND ORGASM? DO YOU ENJOY BEING WATCHED?

Capricorn likes to take his time having sex and delves into a wide range of practices, including bondage and dominance and submission. As a result it is a very important part of the sexual experience for him to observe his partner's reactions. He is quite comfortable being watched as well.

The Big "O"

HOW DO YOU REACH AN ORGASM AND HOW OFTEN?

For Capricorn, who puts a lot of effort into foreplay leading up to climax, that final moment can be brought by a full range of methods and any combination, oral, anal, or manual sex acts.

"Primarily through masturbation as well as with oral sex and anal sex."

"Orgasm happens during all types of sex, not just one specific way."

"Both oral and having my partner masturbate me."

WHAT'S YOUR FAVORITE POSITION?

He says, "any sex is the best position," and he'll accommodate his partner's preference but he does have a special fondness for "69."

"I like '69' for fellatio. Otherwise, I like to lie on my back with my legs on his shoulders, or vice versa. That way I can look at him and kiss and suck all at once."

"Let's see, I like him being on top, me being on top . . . I like them all."

SOME PEOPLE ARE CONCERNED ABOUT BRINGING A PARTNER TO CLIMAX BEFORE HAVING AN ORGASM. OTHERS STRIVE TO REACH ORGASM TOGETHER. WHICH IS TRUE FOR YOU?

Capricorn is a very controlled personality in all aspects of his life, including sex. He strives to time his orgasm to coincide with his partner's or he holds back until his lover climaxes.

"I prefer either together or my partner first, because I get tired after I orgasm and in fairness to my lover, I do not want to be inattentive."

"I love to have it at the same time, but I lean more to pleasing my partner first."

"Prefer together or him before me."

"I like to bring my partner to orgasm first."

"It varies, but mostly I like getting him off before I cum."

ARE YOU VOCAL DURING SEX?

From moaning to making considerable sound, Capricorn lets his lover know how satisfied he is feeling.

"I can be very vocal if I feel uninhibited."

A MEMORY

"I was with two guys who did about everything you could think of to me, except harming me. They both just took over and made love to me at the same time for hours. The setting itself was very sexy, with dimmed lights and candles lit, soft slow music playing, and incense in the air."

AFTER SEX WHAT DO YOU LIKE TO DO?

Capricorn is pretty flexible about his post-sex behaviors. He will want to cuddle for a while, and perhaps take a shower. After that, the rest depends upon the time of day.

"If it is in the a.m. it is a lovely start to the day. If it is in the p.m. we fall asleep together."

"Shower together and eat a meal and then lie down to relax or sleep."

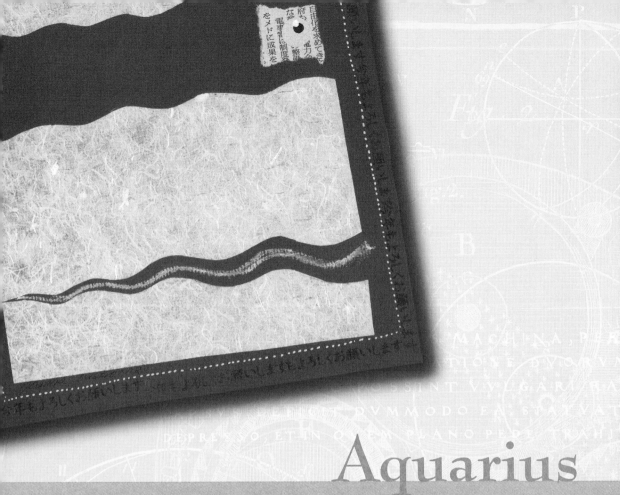

Aquarius
THE WATER BEARER
January 20 through February 18

Seduce my mind and you can have my

body. Find my soul and I'm yours forever."

—Lilly Nomad

AIR SIGN AQUARIUS is the Sign of brotherhood. Aquarians are diplomatic, friendly, and generous. They find intelligence sexy and they're great communicators. Ruler of the ankles and circulation, sexy talk and anything that gets the blood moving, sports, a work out, or a massage, puts Aquarius in the mood for sex.

He says: "Sex with the man I love is like seeing God and gives answers to almost all the impossible questions."

The Aquarius Man
in His Own Words

"I was at a bathhouse with a group of seven anonymous guys. We were in the cloudy steam room. The walls were dripping. We were all engaged in touching each other and acts of sex. Between the dim light and the heavy steam I couldn't see much at all, but the sounds and touches were exciting. It was great consensual sex, not too aggressive, hot and romantic with the sweaty, moist, clean smell of men. They all came on me in the end."

Attraction and Dating an Aquarius

WHAT ATTRACTS YOU TO SOMEONE?

He is very attentive to a man's physique, especially attracted by a man's lips. Aquarius is an Air Sign, and all Air Signs are concerned with communication so intellectual ability and awareness about what is going on in the world are sexy to him. In fact, even a man who just isn't his type physically will capture Aquarius's attention if he is well mannered, intelligent, and a lively conversationalist.

"Confidence, goodness, innate sexiness, kissable lips, intense eyes. I am a sucker for great pecs, a good attitude, men who feel that they don't have to prove anything."

"Tall, athletic, muscular, a successful professional, intelligent, well educated, funny, easygoing, and sexy mouth or lips."

"A person's lips, the unique characteristics of an individual, honesty, intimacy, awareness; the way they talk, a person's lines, and the way they own them or their body communication."

WHAT MIGHT TURN YOU OFF?

Aquarius is the Sign of the diplomat. He can go anywhere and meet anyone and behave in an appropriate way. As a result, bad manners as well as poor hygiene are a definite turn off.

"Bad manners, unhygienic, cruel, snobby, feminine."

"Bad behavior, bad manners, bad teeth and breath."

"Bad attitudes, denseness, fat, lying, games."

MEMORIES

"Lying on the sand dunes hearing the ocean crashing around us, and the smell of sex mixing with the salt air, and feeling the sun beating down on our hot bodies."

"Having sex in a dorm room with a straight guy while a party was going on in the next room. We burned some incense, put on some music, and had very aggressive sex. I remember lots of violent thrusting and yet we were trying to be very quiet."

WHAT DO YOU ENJOY DOING ON A DATE?

Regardless of what else comprises an evening with Aquarius, he always mentions the importance of talking. He loves to discuss local as well as international events. For Aquarius the most erogenous zone is unmistakably the brain.

"Movies, dinner, talking, connecting with mutual interests, museums, sex, cooking for the person, music interests."

"Going for dinner or having coffee, or simply talking on the phone, or meeting face to face."

"Dinner, good conversation, kiss, flirt."

"Dinner, drinks, talking, dancing, walking, having sex, sleeping with someone."

ARE YOU FLIRTATIOUS?

Aquarius is charming and talkative. He has a way of making the other person feel truly attended to, really listened to. It is this quality, more than anything else that he does or says, that makes him come across as flirtatious.

"Yes, I am very flirtatious, unknowingly."

"Very, it is one of my better qualities."

ARE YOU JEALOUS?

If he sees his lover deeply engrossed in conversation with someone else, he will be jealous, because for him words and ideas are sexy. He feels any in-depth conversation could lead to a sexual encounter.

"Yes, to an extent, only when there is distrust."

"Often, unfortunately, irrationally."

"Not extreme, but more than the average person."

HOW DO YOU FEEL ABOUT PUBLIC DISPLAYS OF AFFECTION?

Public displays are great in the proper place. After all, Aquarius is the Sign of diplomacy and he does not want to do anything that might be perceived as offensive.

A FANTASY

"I imagine that my partner comes home with one of the straight cute guys from the neighborhood, saying 'He wants to know if we can take care of him sexually.' My partner and I take turns giving him head. And then this straight man spreads the word to his friends, so we can take care of all of them."

"It depends where we are. In Provincetown, Massachusetts, I am very comfortable. In my hometown, I need to be careful of homophobes."

"I am comfortable with them to a point, my surroundings make a difference."

"All for it, so long as it is about the affection, genuinely, and not about showing off."

Sexual Attitudes and Behaviors

HOW OFTEN DO YOU THINK ABOUT SEX AND HOW OFTEN PER WEEK DO YOU WANT TO HAVE SEX?

Interest in sex for Aquarius is motivated by sexy conversation. There are usually several times in the course of the week when images turn his thoughts to sex, and if possible he would enjoy getting together with a partner four or five times weekly, if not every day.

HOW LONG DO YOU LIKE TO SPEND HAVING SEX AND HOW MUCH OF THAT TIME IS FOREPLAY? DO YOU ENJOY QUICKIES?

As a rule, he does not want to be rushed, enjoying taking time at foreplay. But foreplay for him includes the intellectual stimulation and anticipation that comes from hot sex talk. Quickies are enjoyable on occasion.

"I prefer one to two hours for sex with one half hour to an hour of foreplay and quickies are okay at times."

"For real true sex, making love, the amount of time is immaterial. Quickies sure."

"I would like to spend hours. It is usually twenty to forty minutes. I enjoy quickies, but prefer long foreplay."

"My preference is one to three hours, with about half of that on foreplay. Quickies yes."

FANTASIES

"My favorite fantasies involve men who are very masculine and muscular, like truckers. I see them as feeling lonely, staying in some roadside motel, with no chance for release, other than watching TV porn and using their own right hand."

"I come across a group of skateboarders near a freeway overpass. They have lots of tattoos and piercings. We sit around drinking some beers and smoking some weed. Casually one of them suggests giving him a blow job and I wind up doing the whole group."

WHAT TIME OF DAY DO YOU PREFER TO HAVE SEX?

Time of day is irrelevant to Aquarius. Morning, noon, or night, turn him on and he's good to go.

HOW OFTEN PER WEEK DO YOU MASTURBATE?

This is a man who gets turned on by conversation, for whom the brain is a sex organ. As a result he isn't likely to masturbate very often unless he's participating in phone sex or using pornography as stimulus.

HOW LONG DO YOU WANT TO KNOW SOMEONE BEFORE GETTING SEXUAL?

When Aquarius is attracted to someone, it doesn't take him long to act on his desire to become sexual and if no intimate relationship develops, he'll strive to remain friends.

"For quickies, one minute is okay. For a relationship, one to two weeks."

"I don't have to know someone at all to have sex with him."

"It makes no difference as long as they are nice."

"I tend to get sexual right at the beginning. If the sex isn't any good, the relationship won't continue on an intimate level but we can just be friends."

WHAT'S YOUR ATTITUDE TOWARD CASUAL SEX?

Casual sex is okay but not great because all it can do is satisfy a physical urge. It cannot satisfy the Aquarian's primary sex organ, his brain.

"It is okay, as long as I had my mind set on just sex and have no emotional attachment."

"Casual sex is fine, though often boring, and not worth all the effort."

"It's fine, you just have to be careful physically and emotionally."

A MEMORY

"For the first time tonight I was turned down. He wanted to know me better before engaging in sex. He did not even want to cuddle. He said he wouldn't have any self-control. He touched my heart and earned such respect from me."

DO YOU BELIEVE IN MONOGAMY?

He does, though it may not be easy. First and foremost, a lover must continue to hold his interest. When his mind wanders, so will his body.

"Yes, I do, however I don't think that it is necessarily forever nor is it for everyone. I believe that you just let relationships evolve."

"Yes, but it is a difficult thing to maintain as a gay man."

"I believe in true love and monogamy. If I love someone I do not have sex with another person because that would destroy my relationship."

"Absolutely. When I am in love I have no physical interest in anyone other than that person."

"Yes, definitely . . . in theory."

DOES SEX HAVE A SPIRITUAL SIGNIFICANCE FOR YOU?

Aquarius seeks sensation in all aspects of life, certainly through sex. Therefore, many Aquarians see sex as primarily physical. Only when he feels he has found

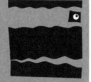

A FANTASY

"I have fantasies involving bare feet, meeting a hunky guy in flip-flops while I am at the supermarket. We go back to his place, he kisses me on both cheeks and leads me to his bedroom. We undress very slowly, his sandals still on. As he lies on the bed I take off one flip-flop and begin to suck each toe, one at a time, as he jerks off and cums. He has never had his toes sucked before."

a truly loving relationship, and he lets down some of his guard, does he acknowledge a spiritual side to sex.

"No, just physical pleasure, relaxation, however it could be spiritual if I were to find my significant other."

"It is when you become aware of your partner's pleasure more than your own."

"Yes, when two souls unite, even for casual sex. It is an exchange of energies and should never be taken lightly or for granted."

"Connecting with anyone is spiritual, no matter how brief or extended that connection is. It becomes a part of one's body map."

"Sex with the man I love is like seeing God and gives answers to almost all the impossible questions."

ARE YOU COMFORTABLE INITIATING SEXUAL ACTIVITIES?

Without reservation, Aquarius is comfortable talking about sex and willingly makes the first move.

"Yes, I am so creative, but I don't always want to be the aggressor."

HOW DO YOU COMMUNICATE TO YOUR PARTNER YOUR SEXUAL WANTS AND NEEDS?

Aquarius, an Air Sign, is a good communicator. He is comfortable expressing his sexual desires both verbally and with body language.

"Both, but mainly I have to spell it out for him with words."

"Mostly gestures, early in a relationship words are necessary. If you truly know someone, words are unnecessary. Gestures and facial expression tell all."

DO YOU THINK OF YOURSELF AS BEING IN THE MAINSTREAM SEXUALLY, MORE EXPERIMENTAL, OR OPEN TO ANYTHING?

He is a fairly experimental lover, into anal sex, as top or bottom, gets a kick out of using food, wearing leather or latex, ménage à trois, and voyeurism. For toys he loves dildoes. He may not have tried electricity yet, but he'd enjoy it. The most open Aquarians are into water sports but seldom into heavy sadomasochism.

"I am definitely experimental, I may not be up for 'anything' but I do love to try new ways and new things."

In his fantasy life, he envisions aggressive scenes with multiple partners and activities ranging from double penetration to rape.

HOW DO YOU DEMONSTRATE AFFECTION FOR YOUR PARTNER?

Here too, Aquarius demonstrates his skill as a communicator. He is willing to help solve problems or merely offer an attentive ear. In addition, he strives to be helpful in sharing responsibilities at home.

"Communicate with him, bring him small things that I know he would like, sharing inside jokes."

"Sending cards, flowers, little gifts, and telling him I love him."

"Holding doors, kissing, holding hands, doing the unexpected."

"Showing interest and kindness."

> ## A FANTASY
>
> "Gang rape with cowboys, leather daddy fetishes, bondage, threesomes, bestiality. I want sex with some wild rock star, a mechanic, a police officer, straight guys, or with a doctor in his office. I imagine sex while getting a tattoo, being pierced, while having a massage, or at work. Sometimes my fantasies are set outside, at the beach, or at a bathhouse."

The Five Senses

HOW IMPORTANT TO YOU IS THE SEXUAL ENVIRONMENT?

Once his brain is focused on sex, what he wants is intense sexual sensation. This may come from foreplay, from involvement with fetishes or sex toys, but the sexual experience is rarely about the environment. It should not be rank and disgusting, but overall the setting is of very little consequence.

"Not very important, sometimes a little dirt is great, just not filthy. Rotten food and bugs are a definite no."

"Cleanliness is important, but the surroundings are never as important as my partner is."

"I would say that it is somewhat important, clean, comfortable, soft, cool temperature."

"I like it to be dark, clean, odorless, cool."

A MEMORY

"It was a night when my partner and I decided to pick up a hustler and bring him home for a threesome. I enjoyed watching my partner having sex with the other guy. He was really getting into it. His vocalizing, moans, the way they switched off back and forth, the smell of sex all filling the room were an incredible turn-on. What made it even more exciting was seeing my partner act slightly aggressive with the other guy, forcing his penis into the hustler's mouth."

WHERE DO YOU LIKE TO HAVE SEX?

Aquarius is a bit of a thrill seeker. He probably invented the mile-high club.

"Definitely public places, outdoors, in the car."

"All places, exhibitionism runs high here."

"In the beginning at home, if committed, anywhere."

"I have only had sex indoors but would like to do it outdoors."

WHAT PUTS YOU IN THE MOOD FOR SEX?

His partner's willingness is often all that it takes. But beyond that, it is important to remember that Aquarius is an Air Sign and that his most dominant sex organ is the brain. Almost anything that he hears, therefore, from sensual music to erotic movies to sexy conversation will get him set for sex.

"Whenever I see my partner looking provocative."

"Sexy movies, romantic settings, candles and aroma therapy, bathing together."

"Manly scent, porno, catching a glimpse of my partner, touching the nape of my neck, dancing."

"Touch, if someone can touch me and kiss me the right way, then they have won me over."

"It's the person I want to have sex with that puts me in the mood. Just being with him . . . that is my ultimate turn on."

"Good music, a workout, listening to my lover's breath."

WHAT'S YOUR ATTITUDE TOWARD PORNOGRAPHY?

He has something of a take-it-or-leave-it attitude toward porn. Aquarius seeks to feel things intensely. When he is with a partner, pornography is just distracting. When he is alone it can be stimulating, but it takes good pornography to turn him on.

"It is okay, I would rather be doing it than watching it."

"It has its purpose. It has excited me. I like it."

"When not in a relationship it is great. When committed to another I have no interest."

"I use it for masturbation. It is fun at times."

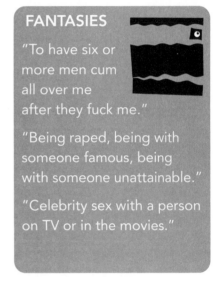

FANTASIES

"To have six or more men cum all over me after they fuck me."

"Being raped, being with someone famous, being with someone unattainable."

"Celebrity sex with a person on TV or in the movies."

HOW MUCH CUDDLING DO YOU ENJOY, ASIDE FROM SEX?

Aquarius isn't known as a particularly touchy-feely Sign. But he views himself as very into cuddling. It seems that in the right place and at the right time, he can be very affectionate.

"As much as I can get, with just the right guy. I find cuddling more personal than sex itself."

"A lot. More than sex."

"More cuddling, sex is great, but cuddling is so sweet and intimate too."

"During movies or at the park and kissing in public, yes. A little spooning after sex, not cuddling all the time."

"Not too much, because it will definitely turn into sex."

HOW TACTILE AND HOW ORAL ARE YOU?

As he seeks sensation in all aspects of sex, he wants to touch and be touched with hands and tongue in all erogenous areas.

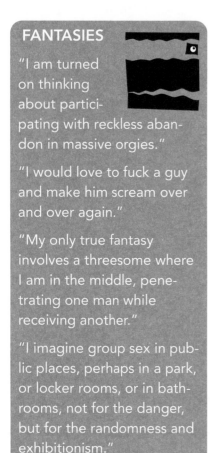

FANTASIES

"I am turned on thinking about participating with reckless abandon in massive orgies."

"I would love to fuck a guy and make him scream over and over again."

"My only true fantasy involves a threesome where I am in the middle, penetrating one man while receiving another."

"I imagine group sex in public places, perhaps in a park, or locker rooms, or in bathrooms, not for the danger, but for the randomness and exhibitionism."

"I like to fondle, scratch his back, feel him up."

"I am very tactile, I love his chest hair."

"Very tactile, touch is important, but sometimes I don't like to be touched all over."

"My tongue is probably my most sensitive body part."

"I enjoy everything tactile and oral, giving and receiving."

"I love it all, very, very oral, kissing and licking, yeah!"

WHAT SEX ACTS DO YOU LIKE MOST AND LEAST?

He enjoys all mainstream sexual acts, from kissing to mutual masturbation and oral sex plus a fair range of experimental behaviors. Anal sex may not be to his liking.

"I love oral sex. There really isn't a favorite, I like some things more with different people."

"I truly have no favorites. What I like best is whatever is turning us both on at the same time and I can't think of any acts that I like least."

"I love kissing, fondling, receiving rimming. I don't enjoy receiving anal sex."

"My favorite is oral and giving anal sex, with poppers of course. I don't like getting anal sex or nipple pinching."

"Favorites: oral sex, giving anal sex, mutual masturbation, fondling balls and ass. Least: receiving anal."

AS A LOVER, WHAT'S YOUR BEST SKILL?

As part of his desire to feel intensely, Aquarius puts all his energy into the moment. As a result, he is quite skillful with his hands and mouth.

"I'm very good at rimming."

"I have been complimented on my kissing and touch many times."

"Great ass, very passionate kisser, massaging, stroking. How I give oral sex."

"I give great head, and I am never too tense to get fucked, but I am still as tight as a guitar string."

WHAT SMELLS AND TASTES ON YOUR PARTNER DO YOU ENJOY?

It's all part of the range of sensory stimuli that get Aquarius hot, smells and tastes of his lover, clean, a bit salty, with and without colognes.

"I like all of his smells. Personal smell is like a drug for me. I particularly like the taste of his sweat."

"I like the smell of his skin, but not right after a shower. I really like his natural body smells, the light scent of his cologne, light body aroma. For tastes, light sweat."

"I enjoy the smell of his cologne and both the smell and taste of his genitals. I like the natural tastes all over his body."

"To start, I like the smell of his cologne and then crotch musk and sweet skin. I love a clean but not soapy smell. For tastes, I love the naturalness of clean skin and the soft sweet taste of the genital region."

A MEMORY

"My favorite sex memory was with a great guy who was leaving town the next day to work for the summer. He came over to my place to say 'Good-bye.' He was wearing a baseball cap that he knew I especially liked. As soon as he got in the door, he leaned back against the wall and took out his cock. I blew him right there in the hallway. He kept his clothes on throughout. He bent down several times and kissed me passionately."

FOR SOME PEOPLE THE TASTE OF THEIR PARTNER'S CUM IS UNPLEASANT. IF THAT'S TRUE FOR YOU, WHAT DO YOU DO ABOUT THE TASTE?

Health concerns aside, Aquarius rarely has any difficulty with the taste of a man's cum; on the contrary, he usually revels in it.

"That's not true for me, I use it as lube for my orgasm."

"What do I do about the taste? Nothing. I enjoy his orgasm in my mouth. I like to swallow, and sometimes I like him to cum on me."

"Taste is usually good, diet plays a large role in how pleasurable the taste will be. If I'm in a committed relationship, I swallow or rub his cum. An old Chinese woman told me it is great for your skin, to rub it on your face. She looked twenty-five to thirty years younger than her true age."

"I like the taste but I haven't had a serious enough relationship to swallow. I rub it all over my face and body."

A MEMORY

"It was a random encounter. I met two men, who were a committed couple, on the street. They were both tall and good looking; in fact, one of them was a model. They invited me to join them in their hotel room for sex. What followed next included lots of touching, exploring, cuddling, and multiple positions. We all ejaculated at the same time, a very rare and difficult thing to do."

DO YOU ENJOY WATCHING YOUR PARTNER DURING SEX AND ORGASM? DO YOU ENJOY BEING WATCHED?

Noting that for him sexual excitement begins in the brain and that he seeks sensory stimulation in all areas, it follows that he thoroughly enjoys observing his lover as well as being watched by him.

"What is the point otherwise?"

"Yes, very much, stimulating to stare into each other's eyes during sex."

"I enjoy my partner looking at me during sex, but not if he isn't participating."

"Yes, though I am somewhat self-conscious."

The Big "O"

HOW DO YOU REACH AN ORGASM AND HOW OFTEN?

Aquarius cums every time he has sex, at least once. When he is very turned on, he is likely to climax almost at once through mutual masturbation. The second time may result from a combination of oral sex and anal intercourse.

WHAT'S YOUR FAVORITE POSITION?

True to his love of variety and sensation, there is no best position for Aquarius.

"I like them all but especially when my lover lies across my chest with all his weight and I have my hands on his butt."

"There is no best. Different partners in different positions. I like being in a sling with them on top or from the back."

SOME PEOPLE ARE CONCERNED ABOUT BRINGING A PARTNER TO CLIMAX BEFORE HAVING AN ORGASM. OTHERS STRIVE TO REACH ORGASM TOGETHER. WHICH IS TRUE FOR YOU?

Most often, Aquarius wants his partner to cum first. Watching his partner's orgasm heightens his own excitement, especially if his partner is fairly vocal when cumming.

"I try to bring my partner to orgasm first."

"I don't want to have an orgasm before my partner. Their orgasm is what gives me mine."

"Together is nice, or very near together, although sometimes it's nice to do it separately so the focus is completely on that person."

"I try to reach it together but have more concern about my partner."

ARE YOU VOCAL DURING SEX?

As an Air Sign, Aquarius is very comfortable with communication. During sex he is vocal, moderately to very much so, depending upon the response of his partner.

AFTER SEX WHAT DO YOU LIKE TO DO?

Aquarius has a reputation for being a bit detached in many settings. After sex, when he feels emotionally close to his partner, it is important to him to take some time to linger, to cuddle.

"After sex, that is the best time, the most intimate. All defenses are down, just lying in bed is the most satisfying thing."

"Shower, cuddle, sleep."

A MEMORY

"After having lunch in my bedroom at a table set up beautifully just for the occasion, we disrobed and kissed a lot. My partner stretched out on the bed. I sat on his cock. I slowly started to pump up and down, breathing hard and heavy. I felt my insides expand, and we both screamed as we came at the same time. After we finished I was still mounting him with him still rock hard inside me."

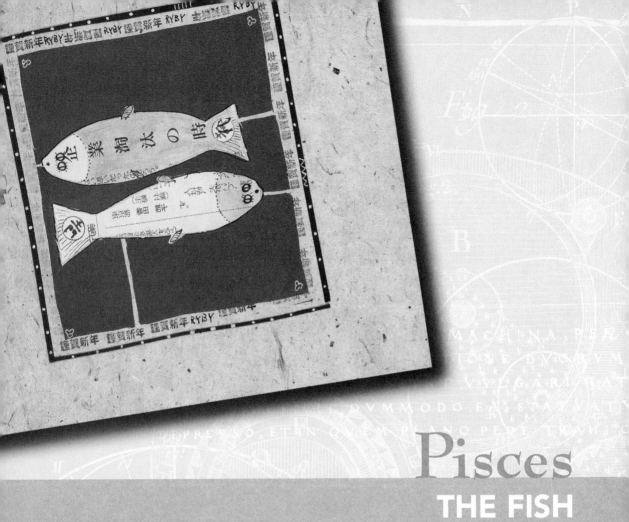

Pisces

THE FISH

February 19 through March 20

WATER SIGN PISCES is very sexual, psychic, and imaginative. They make wonderful writers, storytellers, and actors and have innate healing abilities taking them into the fields of medicine and counseling. Ruler of the feet, which are usually very well formed, a foot massage will turn their thoughts to sex.

He says: "My lover was wearing a leather jockstrap. I put a huge dildo in his ass and made him cum with full ejaculation by manipulating the dildo."

"This is the miracle that happens every time to those who really love; the more they give, the more they possess."

—Rainer Maria Rilke

The Pisces Man
in His Own Words

A MEMORY

"A beautiful man approached me in the restroom of a public park. I had run in there to get out of an unexpected extremely heavy rainstorm. Against the sound of wind and rain beating on the steel roof, I gave him a blow job, that he later described as awesome. Since we were alone, after the act, he kissed me so passionately, that I trembled. We never exchanged names."

Attraction and Dating a Pisces

WHAT ATTRACTS YOU TO SOMEONE?

The twelfth Sign of the zodiac, Pisces, has characteristics of all other eleven Signs. So, when it comes to identifying what it takes to attract his attention, his list of attributes is long and varied. He is attracted to men who are relatively small, not too skinny, and yet masculine. Physical characteristics are important to him as well as a general sense of decorum.

"I like men who know what they want and what they are doing in bed. I want to sleep with men who keep safety as a priority in their lovemaking. Cleanliness and a good personality are also essential."

"I notice a man's lips and hands. I like a man who is in shape, active in life, and a kid at heart. Sexy arms and a nicely developed chest are a plus, as are beautiful feet."

"The first thing I notice is a nice build, a cute face and then, to hold my interest, a great sense of humor."

"A good-looking man with a nice ass, cock, chest, and not too skinny. A man with some meat on him who loves to get fucked, likes to kiss, hug, and have his cock sucked, ass rimmed, a man who loves being touched."

WHAT MIGHT TURN YOU OFF?

Pisces is not aggressive by nature and will be turned of by a man who is argumentative, rude or generally bad mannered. Physical characteristics that turn him off include being extremely thin, extremely heavy, having overly developed muscles, or paying little attention to hygiene. In the big picture, however, a man's looks are far less important to Pisces than his behavior.

WHAT DO YOU ENJOY DOING ON A DATE?

He enjoys a traditional range of evening out activities, such as going to a restaurant, attending a movie, or going to the theater. He also likes entertaining at home. One thing that always pleases him is music. A good sound system at home may be as satisfactory as attending a concert. And any date or evening together should certainly include sex.

"I love having someone come over to my place, have a few beers, and listen to music. It's always good to talk. I enjoy going out to a neighborhood bar and then coming home and having sex, or going out to dinner and having sex afterward."

"A nice dinner, theater or a movie, then followed up with some hot sex."

"Being silly at fun places, like arcades or fun parks, eating, walking and talking about our passions, participating in the arts—shows, movies, concerts."

"I am equally satisfied staying at home or going out to dinner, to movies, or to a bar."

"A dinner and talking over coffee and tea, maybe a movie. I am not into loud scenes."

ARE YOU FLIRTATIOUS?

Pisces has a healing presence, a quality that attracts people to him. In fact, he is decidedly flirtatious, though he may not think of his behavior as anything but being good-natured.

"I tend to put out a vibe, wittingly or unwittingly."

"Yes, very, sometimes unintentionally."

"I am very flirtatious, all the time."

"I like to be coy and subtle with my flirting."

ARE YOU JEALOUS?

Pisces has a vulnerable streak. He may not always be jealous, but that feeling can be triggered, particularly if he is with a man who doesn't reveal his feelings openly.

"I can be jealous sometimes, but I get over it soon enough."

"I can be slightly jealous, but I try not to let it control me."

HOW DO YOU FEEL ABOUT PUBLIC DISPLAYS OF AFFECTION?

Pisces is something of a performer and likes attention. He is, therefore, quite comfortable with public displays. At the same time, however, he has a sensitive and empathetic nature so he is concerned about the feelings of others.

"Under the right circumstance they are fine, but I do not approve of gay or straight people who feel they have to go overboard to make a point. I like to respect other people's spaces as well."

"Public displays of affection are fine, however, I am conscious of others around me and do not want to offend. On the other hand, I do not apologize for my feelings."

"Very good as long as we are among gay people or in a place such as San Francisco."

"I am fine with them as long as the displays are simple and do not go so far that you really need a room."

FANTASIES

"I imagine having sex with two guys. I am giving oral sex to the one, while the other guy would be giving me a good fuck up my ass."

"Sleeping with a totally hot stranger and sometimes not even getting a name. In other fantasies I am with multiple partners, such as three ways with boyfriends and hot older men."

"I have no control of the situation and I am with more than one person."

"The primary image is big dicks, nice bodies, big pecs. Sometimes I use videos that have lots of oral sex going on."

"Images include unexpected group sex, doing it with the naughty pizza boy, incest sex with my brothers and with friends and our dads."

Sexual Attitudes and Behaviors

HOW OFTEN DO YOU THINK ABOUT SEX AND HOW OFTEN PER WEEK DO YOU WANT TO HAVE SEX?

Pisces has an active imagination and sexual images are part of his thought pattern on a daily basis. With a new partner he wants sex daily. Over time he is satisfied with five encounters weekly.

A MEMORY

"My boyfriend is an over six-foot-tall gymnast in great shape. When he has just finished up his practicing, he is sexually charged. One time we drove to the coast and got undressed by the water and we made love near the sea. I still remember the fresh ocean smells."

HOW LONG DO YOU LIKE TO SPEND HAVING SEX AND HOW MUCH OF THAT TIME IS FOREPLAY? DO YOU ENJOY QUICKIES?

On average he enjoys spending an hour for sex. Foreplay is a real variable with Pisces. At most, he wants to spend thirty minutes because he prefers to have several rounds, cumming multiple times. Quickies are only okay on occasion.

"Amount of time on foreplay depends on how much time my partner and I have to devote to the encounter. Sometimes skipping the foreplay and getting to the main course is just fine. I like more foreplay with new partners if it is convenient."

"I enjoy quickies with people I do not know, and two hours with people I know well."

"I like to spend a couple of hours with a partner, but quickies sometimes have to suffice."

"Generally I like one hour. Quickies, seldom, but they are enjoyable."

WHAT TIME OF DAY DO YOU PREFER TO HAVE SEX?

He has a slight preference for late afternoon, evenings, and nighttime, meaning that mornings are about the only time he may not be completely enthusiastic. In the big picture, Pisces will make himself available at any time.

HOW OFTEN PER WEEK DO YOU MASTURBATE?

He masturbates on average five times a week.

HOW LONG DO YOU WANT TO KNOW SOMEONE BEFORE GETTING SEXUAL?

Pisces is extremely intuitive. He acts on instinct in determining when to begin a physical relationship, but it seldom takes very long.

"Ideally if the other person is okay with it, I like to get to it as quickly as possible. I have met some people that I can have incredible sex with and get along with great in bed, but have no interest in maintaining other types of relationships. If this is something that I think might lead to a significant relationship, then I would probably want to get to know the person a little bit more before just jumping in the sack."

"Depends on the energy, vibe, or conversation. Sometimes no time at all."

"At least a couple of weeks. Foreplay and kissing can happen in a few days."

"Right away is okay, as long as it is safe."

> **A MEMORY**
>
> "We went to Provincetown, Massachusetts. I remember several sexual encounters there, some that took place in my room on my waterbed and others lying in his bed. We also did it on a blanket in the woods and then on the beach at night. I remember the scent of his cologne, the sounds that he made during sex, the smell of his body, and especially his clean asshole, and then rimming his ass and finishing up with anal sex."

WHAT'S YOUR ATTITUDE TOWARD CASUAL SEX?

He has no illusions about anonymous sex. It can be fun and overall it is fine, but is of limited satisfaction. He doesn't consider oral sex to be unsafe.

"If done safely, fine, but I don't do it when I am in a relationship."

"Casual sex is fine as long as it is safe, but knowing a person well makes for better sex."

"It's fine once in a while. I love sucking cock and getting sucked."

"It is totally okay, but it doesn't fulfill me the way sex with a man I know better can."

DO YOU BELIEVE IN MONOGAMY?

Pisces has traditional values and is by nature a spiritual person. The most comfortable relationships for him, in keeping with his general philosophy, are therefore, monogamous.

"Yes, the only way to love is monogamy."

"Yes, why be in a relationship if you are not going to be monogamous?"

"I like to fool around, but if I find the right person I would not cheat on him at all."

"Yes, that situation is my ideal."

A MEMORY

"My boyfriend, he was very young, about twenty years old, made love to me for four hours. I think I came five times, sometimes without his touching me. Over time I taught him to become a total bottom."

DOES SEX HAVE A SPIRITUAL SIGNIFICANCE FOR YOU?

Pisces is not necessarily religious by nature, but he is definitely spiritual. He is comfortable getting in touch with his feelings and the strong bond that sex creates for him with another man is spiritual.

"Yes, it can create a deep connection with the right person."

"Definitely, sex is a physical and spiritual connection between two souls, a partaking in one of the greatest experiences of life."

"Yes, to give yourself to another person is very spiritual."

"Yes, I try not to have sex on Sundays."

ARE YOU COMFORTABLE INITIATING SEXUAL ACTIVITIES?

Pisces is the most psychic Sign in the zodiac. This man can read another person's responses very well, so he is quite at ease opening the subject of sexuality without fear of rejection.

HOW DO YOU COMMUNICATE TO YOUR PARTNER YOUR SEXUAL WANTS AND NEEDS?

Pisces is a sensitive Sign, not overly assertive by nature. As a result, when he wants to make his sexual desires known, he relies mostly on subtle sound and body language.

"I am into the physical act with very little verbal communication, other than moans and groans."

DO YOU THINK OF YOURSELF AS BEING IN THE MAINSTREAM SEXUALLY, MORE EXPERIMENTAL, OR OPEN TO ANYTHING?

Pisces is an experimental lover, open to anal sex, usually topping, and dominance and submission. He enjoys wearing leather, underwear, is open to sex with multiple partners, including orgies, and having sex in public places. Pisces, the Sign that rules the feet, may have a fetish for them. He is also likely to enjoy using hot wax and participating in water sports. When it comes to sex toys, his interest is primarily limited to dildoes.

In addition to images that reflect his range of sexual behaviors, his fantasies frequently include specific places, a setting in the woods, in water, or on some kind of stage set. The activities are straightforward, oral and anal sex, though often fairly aggressive.

> **A FANTASY**
>
> "I fantasize making love in a natural setting, as close to nature as possible, near water, maybe sex under a waterfall. I see myself with a tall man or better yet, an Olympic gymnast. My biggest desire is making love to my boyfriend under water, like mermen."

HOW DO YOU DEMONSTRATE AFFECTION FOR YOUR PARTNER?

Pisces is sensitive to his partner's feelings. He is a good listener, a helpful partner and he loves to buy romantic gifts, small tokens of affection. He is apt to purchase Christmas gifts in July if he comes across something that he knows his partner will adore.

"Making lunch before he goes to work, a back rub when he has had a hard day."

"By being there for him, by listening to him."

"I am thoughtful and conversational, and if there is some special need or desire, I try to fill it for my partner."

"I am a grateful person, big with the thanks."

"Spontaneous acts of kindness, love, and giving."

"Small gifts, trying to make him happy by cooking, cleaning, shopping, gifts."

The Five Senses

●●●

HOW IMPORTANT TO YOU IS THE SEXUAL ENVIRONMENT?

Beyond cleanliness and the use of candles, Pisces does not claim to find the sexual setting overly important. However, he does have a fundamentally romantic nature, and setting the stage with flowers, fresh sheets, perhaps incense, or soft music will surely intensify his mood.

"It is important, but the person is more important."

"Cleanliness is good and I like to be able to see everything, so good light or candles matter to me."

"As long as it is not disgusting, I am okay."

WHERE DO YOU LIKE TO HAVE SEX?

His favorite location is in the bedroom on a comfortable bed. Beyond that, being a Water Sign, he enjoys having sex with water nearby, whether he is in a tent by a stream, on the beach at night, or in a car with the rain beating down.

"One of my favorite places is in a tent in the great outdoors. Hot tubs and pools are also high on my list."

"Pretty much wherever my partner will do it, but in bed is great."

WHAT PUTS YOU IN THE MOOD FOR SEX?

Pisces is ruled by the planet Neptune, which is all about creating illusions. Pisces can be chameleon-like and adept at assuming roles of all sorts. Preparing for sex with sensual stimuli, such as erotic images in films or porn videos, playing sexy music, and wearing musky colognes put him in the mood.

"Porn, candles, and music."

"Sometimes all it takes is a nice glance from a man that I find attractive."

"Watching porn and talking sexy, liquor, poppers."

"Cuddling, watching porn, talking about sex, lighting candles, being naked."

"Aromas, watching porn videos, wearing sexy slacks, tight jeans or shorts, sexy underwear, a big rock-hard cock."

"Porn can put me in the mood, cuddling and sexy talk always do."

WHAT'S YOUR ATTITUDE TOWARD PORNOGRAPHY?

Pisces is a wonderful actor and enjoys the fantasy of projecting himself into the porn videos that he is watching. Playing them when he is with a partner enables him to broaden the range of his own sexual expression.

"Big turn on, love it, helps with sex."

"I love pornography in moderation. Watching it all the time gets redundant."

"Love it, I love to watch gay videos and jerk off."

"There is nothing wrong with pornography at all. It should be a natural part of sexuality."

> ### A FANTASY
>
> "I imagine sex with a movie star or being in a porno film, being naked with a lot of gay men, being able to cum with my friends, cumming together. I had a committed partner once. I was very much in love with him. He was the one who could make me cum, the only one. I fantasize about that."

HOW MUCH CUDDLING DO YOU ENJOY, ASIDE FROM SEX?

From an occasional touch to a hug, sitting close on the couch, Pisces enjoys the closeness of another man.

"I like it very much, nice way to stay close."

"Cuddling is best when kissing, cuddling at home watching TV is fun. I like lots of cuddles."

HOW TACTILE AND HOW ORAL ARE YOU?

Pisces enjoys the full range of touching with his hands, mouth, and tongue.

"Tactile, a lot. I am also very oral and enjoy rimming, kissing, oral sex."

"Light touching, little massage can be fun when they are a prelude or part of the main course. I am very oral. I enjoy giving and receiving head, mostly giving because I am so good at it. If the partner is right and the person is clean, then rimming can be great, both giving and receiving. '69' in any capacity is also a favorite."

"A lot, very playful and touchy. I like to suck dick and enjoy some kissing."

"I love to touch his body, his chest, his penis. I love deep kissing, fellatio, and rimming. They are all favorites."

WHAT SEX ACTS DO YOU LIKE MOST AND LEAST?

He likes all mainstream sex acts from fondling to frottage to oral sex. He dislikes acts that cause pain and is not necessarily enthusiastic about anal intercourse. Beyond the standard range of sex behaviors, he also enjoys such things as wearing leather, having multiple partners, and having a foot massage.

"I like giving and receiving head, rimming, '69,' and mutual masturbation. I do not enjoy anal intercourse or bondage."

A MEMORY

"My lover and I were having a picnic and just the surroundings, the quiet, the warmth . . . one thing led to another, and we made love right there on our blanket out in the open. We did not care who might be watching."

"I like anal sex when I am fucking my partner. I do not like getting fucked. I love oral sex receiving and giving."

"My favorites are anal sex, mutual masturbation, fellatio, and kissing. Least favorite? None."

"Kissing and mutual masturbation, oral sex and intercourse are my favorite acts. I can't think of anything I do not like."

"I like anything, kissing, oral sex, anal sex, as long as it does not involve pain."

AS A LOVER, WHAT'S YOUR BEST SKILL?

Pisces has a psychic streak. He knows things without being aware how he knows them. This is true in his sexual behaviors as well. He can sense a partner's desires and he is usually willing to fulfill them. He is a man for all body parts, quite skilled with his hands, body and mouth.

"I give great head and can chew on a man's tit like nobody's business."

"My skills are massages, touching, kissing, and the way that I can contort my body."

"I am good at keeping my man happy and satisfied and always begging for more."

"The best skill I have is being a giving person, and doing what he wants me to do to him"

"Using my tongue all over."

WHAT SMELLS AND TASTES ON YOUR PARTNER DO YOU ENJOY?

Pisces is a passionate Water Sign who enjoys the full range of smells and tastes. Fresh-washed skin, the groin area when it gets sweaty, clean hair, his lover's feet and some colognes are all exciting to him.

"Manly smells, perspiration, and the smell of fresh cum turn me on as well as the taste of perspiration and sweaty balls."

"I like the smell of his skin and cologne, the natural sexual smell he gives off, the smell and taste of his lips."

"Smells: sensual body oils and his private parts. Tastes: fresh sweat."

"I like the smell of a man's ass and the taste of his cock."

A MEMORY

"Just a wonderful time in my car. It was during a thunderstorm, a particularly fierce one, with pouring rain, loud thunder, and brilliant lightning. Aside from that, all my memories of my boyfriend fucking me, at any time, are wonderful."

FOR SOME PEOPLE THE TASTE OF THEIR PARTNER'S CUM IS UNPLEASANT. IF THAT'S TRUE FOR YOU, WHAT DO YOU DO ABOUT THE TASTE?

He may not prefer the taste of cum, though he usually deals with it when in a committed relationship. In casual sexual encounters, he avoids cum.

"I do not usually taste or ingest a partner's cum, I don't think it is safe anymore. Maybe if I were in a committed relationship I would take cum in my mouth."

"I try to swallow and usually lick up some of it if he cums on his stomach."

"I let it go in my mouth and spit it out. With surprise climaxes, sometimes you just have to swallow."

"I let it go where it wants to. If it lands on me, that is okay. I rub it."

"When I was in a committed relationship, I swallowed."

"If he cums in my mouth, I swallow it quickly before tasting it."

DO YOU ENJOY WATCHING YOUR PARTNER DURING SEX AND ORGASM? DO YOU ENJOY BEING WATCHED?

Given that he is something of a performer and likes attention, he enjoys having his lover observe him. Sometimes he becomes so involved in his own feelings that he closes his eyes and wanders off into his own fantasy. Most of the time watching his lover's pleasure is exciting to him.

The Big "O"

MEMORIES

"My lover was wearing a leather jockstrap. I put a huge dildo in his ass and made him cum with full ejaculation by manipulating the dildo."

"The first time I let my new boyfriend poke me in the ass. He has a huge dick so it was no small feat, but I was determined to take it all. I was so sore afterwards."

HOW DO YOU REACH AN ORGASM AND HOW OFTEN?

He reaches orgasm most of the time though it may be somewhat difficult to climax when his partner is masturbating him.

"I cum all the time through intercourse and a combination of anal sex and masturbation."

"Anal sex all the time, sometimes masturbation, more so when I finish myself off."

"With masturbation and anal sex, I orgasm all the time. With oral sex, rarely."

WHAT'S YOUR FAVORITE POSITION?

Most positions satisfy him. He can be quite creative. But his favorite is "69."

"With anal sex, spooning is my favorite."

"I like '69' and also lying side by side."

"Him on top of me, me on top, doggie style."

"'69,' facing side by side."

"My man on his back with his legs in the air."

SOME PEOPLE ARE CONCERNED ABOUT BRINGING A PARTNER TO CLIMAX BEFORE HAVING AN ORGASM. OTHERS STRIVE TO REACH ORGASM TOGETHER. WHICH IS TRUE FOR YOU?

Pisces is so psychic, so tuned in to his partner, that he generally can time his orgasm to coincide with his lover's.

"I like us to orgasm together."

"I strive to reach orgasm with my partner, but by no means is that a necessity."

"Yes this is important to me. I like us to cum together."

"Very concerned to cum together, always strive to bring my partner to orgasm."

"My partner is usually my main concern, then myself, but cumming at the same time is fun when possible."

ARE YOU VOCAL DURING SEX?

Pisces is fairly talkative to start with, but during sex he prefers moans and sounds rather than carrying on much conversation.

"I would say that I am a little vocal . . . mostly with moans and groans."

"Yes, I love to moan, groan, breathe, talk."

"I am a moaner."

AFTER SEX WHAT DO YOU LIKE TO DO?

He may be tired and want to sleep. He might be hungry and want to eat. On occasion he prefers to relax together for a while. In other words, he has no set behavior after sex, with perhaps one exception. He usually likes to take a shower.

"It depends on the circumstances. Usually I just thank the man and leave."

"I like to take a shower, relax, and then maybe do it again."

"Engage in something relaxing with my partner, perhaps have something to eat."

"Shower and go out together."

"Shower first then have a snack."

Sexual Compatibility through the Zodiac

Aries ~ Aries
Two Rams together ~ can they avoid butting heads?

This is way too much fire. It's an ego contest. Whoever wins is the one with the most blessings from above. In bed there's no intrigue. It's slam-bam and neither Aries knows how to broaden the perspective. Though both say they like spending quite a while having sex, thirty minutes to an hour, two Aries together wind up moving way too fast to feel gratified. For better sex, one needs to be more evasive and make the other work harder.

Anytime two of the same Sign form a couple there can be conflict. There is no balance. Because both will be under similar astrological elements, when one Aries is having trouble, in all likelihood the other Aries is as well. He comes home from work saying, "I had the worst day. The guy in the next cubicle is driving me nuts." Partner Aries replies, "Wait 'til I tell you about my day." This is hardly comforting for either. In addition, Aries is apt to be abrupt verbally. No harm intended, but the Aries on the receiving end is easily wounded.

In an Aries/Aries pairing, the greatest likelihood for success occurs if one Aries is seven years or so older than the other. An older partner may be more willing to concede to the other and may be less likely to feel threatened by the other Aries's youthful exuberance and need to make all the rules. The older Aries may not mind pampering the little one. Conversely, younger Aries enjoys being nurtured and indulged.

SUMMARY

Aries is a perpetual little boy, about the age of six. He's old enough to know what he wants and he won't be deterred until he gets it. With two equally headstrong little boys, neither one willing to concede or compromise, there is conflict, not companionship. The sex may be fiery for a while, but it's not likely to be satisfying for long. One reason is that Aries is rather predictable in sexual behavior and wants some outside stimulus to try greater variety. If one of these Aries is willing to assume that responsibility, the relationship can be sustained a while longer.

Aries ~ Taurus
The Ram and the Bull ~ the dust will fly

In the first days, Aries enchants Taurus and life is beautiful. Taurus grows up feeling that he was not loved enough, no matter how much he was loved. Along comes Aries whose behavior consumes Taurus with passionate love. Meanwhile, Aries, longing to be doted on, is gratified by Taurus's total focus.

So what's the problem? Aries is bossy and Taurus will not be told what to do. Ask a Taurus for help, and you get it. Tell a Taurus to help, and you get an argument. Aries wants to be in control and while Taurus is very willing to be second in command, very willing to be supportive, Taurus will not follow orders. When Aries is aggressive, Taurus becomes unyielding. When speedy Aries says, "Let's do it now," slow-moving Taurus asks, "Why, what's the hurry?"

In bed and out, this conflict of style undermines the long-term potential for a successful relationship. Taurus wants to luxuriate in sex, savoring it rather like a seven-course meal. For Aries sex is more like the appetizer or the dessert. Over time, in the bedroom, Aries would be bored to death with Taurus.

Out of the bedroom, Aries's readiness to do things at the drop of a hat runs headlong into Taurus's need to consider an action for a stretch of time before participating. What makes this combination so difficult is the conflict between the fundamental qualities of Aries—assertiveness and risk-taking—versus Taurus's stability, receptivity, and need for security.

SUMMARY

Who's in charge here? Aries, of course. Wait a minute, Taurus won't put up with that. Taurus says, "Don't tell me what to do." But no matter how many times Aries hears this, he keeps on doing it. Aries says, "You're stubborn." Taurus says, "You're selfish." Aries says, "Let's go out." Taurus says, "Let's stay home." Clearly, for these two to have any relationship whatsoever after the initial passion cools, a division of power will be necessary, coupled with greater sensitivity on the part of the Aries and a bit more flexibility on the part of Taurus.

Aries ~ Gemini
The Ram and the Twins ~ endless possibilities

Aries is the Sign of exploration, Gemini the Sign of experimentation. These two ideas are compatible and these Signs are a natural combination. While Gemini might be content to read and think about something, Aries will say, "Come on, let's go out and do it." This enthusiasm is captivating to Gemini.

With Aries what you see is what you get. Gemini, on the other hand is a more complex dual sign. Aries tends to focus on one thing at a time. Gemini is apt to be involved in a dozen things simultaneously. It's part of Gemini's life path to try out many things. Gemini grows bored when life is too settled. Aries keeps Gemini guessing. With a less dynamic partner, Gemini pays inadequate attention, begins to withdraw, and everything falls apart. Aries dynamism and intensity serve to keep Gemini steadfast.

When it comes to sex, Aries and Gemini are also very well matched. Gemini intuitively knows to make Aries put a little more effort into lovemaking. Gemini is a verbal sign and keeps some banter going with Aries, asking questions, slowing the pace. As Aries likes being given sexual directions, it works that Gemini is the natural leader between these two. There is a minor problem but one that can grow over time if Gemini doesn't attend to it. Gemini is better with his hands than with his mouth or lips. Aries is turned on by passionate kissing. For Aries the force in a lover's kiss is proof of love.

SUMMARY

The best thing about these two Signs is their remarkable ability to communicate about an extraordinary range of subjects. Gemini is constantly learning new things and Aries is always up for something different. These two have a relationship that is part brother and part best friend. Jealousy is apt to be a problem. Even though Gemini is a flirt, he is distressed to see his partner behaving flirtatiously and there is no doubt that Aries will do so. To keep their comfortable sex life more interesting, sometimes Aries needs to be the leader and allow Gemini his fantasy of being totally controlled.

Aries ~ Cancer
The Ram with the Crab ~ steam up or sputter out?

Aries is a Fire Sign. Cancer is Water. Together they produce steam, at least for a while. But water drowns fire, and Cancer's emotionalism may extinguish Aries passion. Sustaining a relationship will require consistent effort. Yet relationships between these two are sometimes successful and can be gratifying when each accepts the other's differences.

Aries is a perpetual child and Cancer is the nurturing one. Emotions make Aries decidedly uncomfortable. Cancer is intensely emotional. Aries covers most emotions with anger. An upset Cancer needs to work through the feelings, talk about them to release them. But when Aries wants comforting, Cancer is there, strong and loving, and that wonderful Aries courage provides reassurance when Cancer is upset.

In the bedroom, Aries is ready from the onset. Cancer needs time to work up steam. Sometimes Aries isn't sensitive enough to Cancer's moods and may believe that Cancer doesn't have a strong sex drive. Not true. Cancer is highly sexual.

The preferences of these Signs in bed are also different. Aries is experimental in sexual range, including using costumes and light bondage and such sex toys as dildoes and butt plugs. Cancer is more open, into bondage, dominance and submission, and water sports. On the plus side, both prefer sex in the comfort of their home as neither likes to be observed when having sex. Cancer may love making out in the woods but certainly doesn't want to risk being watched. Sex in a secluded pine forest, or at least in a nearby B&B, will revitalize this couple sexually every time.

SUMMARY

For Cancer, an ideal life is the typical American dream—the single-family house with white picket fence and chicken soup cooking on the stove. Aries may want that house, but certainly doesn't want to be fenced in. Cancer spreads his wings and wants to dominate everything within his sphere. Aries will go looking for any and every way out. Without ever meaning to, Aries will hurt Cancer. Can this work? If Cancer doesn't take everything Aries says personally and Aries strives to be a bit more attentive, it might. Generally, the sex may be steamy, the relationship unstable.

Aries ~ Leo
The Ram and the Lion ~ fire burning bright

Putting these two Signs together is a challenge and, at least in bed, it's great. Sexually Aries and Leo are well matched. Both Signs tend to be experimental in their range of behaviors. They love passionate kissing, feverish embraces, quick sex, as well as longer sessions and pride themselves on the strength of their sex drive.

There are some Aries and Leos who are involved in more extreme sex. Here too they match up quite perfectly in their choice of sexual experimentation, including bondage, dominance and submission, and using food in sex play. The sex toys they enjoy fall into the more traditional range, dildoes, vibrators, and cock rings.

A relationship can work, though it won't be easy. Common ground: both are quick thinking and spontaneous; they like the same sorts of activities. But problems often arise because each may see the other as self-centered. Both Signs thrive on praise, for different reasons. Aries is an insecure Sign and seeks ego gratification in all things. He needs to be told how wonderful he is before he believes it himself. Leo, on the other hand, has a strong ego. He doesn't really need praise but he basks in it. Unfortunately, neither of these Signs gives out quite enough compliments.

Another problem area is that both Aries and Leo are uncomfortable apologizing. Aries virtually chokes on the words "I'm sorry." Leo is almost never wrong. In fact, on those rare occasions when Leo really is wrong, he'll gladly accept the other party's apology.

SUMMARY

Who's in control here? Leo says, "I am," but those are the key words for the Sign of Aries. In other words, if Leo wants to be in charge, he'd better not tell Aries. Leo thinks Aries is egocentric. That's really the pot calling the kettle black. In fact, Aries is like a petulant child. Leo is the imperious ruler. Each of these Fire Signs will provoke the other, make the other jealous, and neither is at all adept at apologizing. Can this work? Absolutely. Will it? That all depends on how two independent and powerful egos decide to negotiate.

Aries ~ Virgo
The Ram and the Virgin ~ passion or punishment?

Getting this relationship started is apt to be awkward. Virgo is attracted to Aries but reticent to reveal feelings and waits for Aries to make the first move. Aries isn't shy but wants encouragement. Virgo can be so poker faced, Aries isn't sure Virgo is interested at all, leading to a stalemate. Once this is overcome, Virgo finds Aries enthusiasm, spontaneity, and openness refreshing. Aries is balanced by the down-to-earth, practical approach of Virgo. Aries is quicker to make a commitment than is Virgo, but once they enter into a monogamous relationship, both Signs are faithful.

Still, the differences are vast as these two do almost everything differently. For example, getting ready for a vacation, Aries says, "Let the road take us where it may." Virgo has at least two sets of maps and wants the route fully plotted before leaving home. Aries overlooks the details, trusting to luck. Virgo is very detail oriented.

Aries can't stand criticism, and love on the part of Virgo is picking lint off the collar of his lover. During sex, Virgo will give instructions—a little to the left, a little to the right, do more of this, do more of that. That's fine in the bedroom, because Aries want to satisfy his lover. Outside the bedroom, the Ram wants the freedom to do as he pleases and being nagged by Virgo is a turn-off. Virgo needs to be less critical and Aries must avoid becoming defensive for this relationship to succeed.

SUMMARY

The attraction is electric and Aries looks at Virgo with adoration. Virgo is equally smitten by Aries's vitality. Aries will always need reaffirmation of love. Conversely, Aries needs to acknowledge Virgo's efforts, his willingness to pitch in and help without being asked. Virgo doesn't demand a pat on the back, but it is appreciated. Aries also enjoys getting small gifts as tokens of affection. While Virgo may be very loving in some regards, buying little trinkets is not high on his list of priorities. These two can't change each other. "Vive la difference" or they will go their separate ways.

Aries ~ Libra
The Ram and the Scales ~ opposites attract and repel

It starts out well. Fire Sign Aries brings passion to an affair with Libra. Air Sign Libra cools things down some, making the sex last a little longer. In bed, passionate kissing comes first. Aries also loves having his head caressed and intense oral sex. Libra will want to satisfy Aries, but is not interested in the same sexual acts. While both enjoy voyeurism and a certain amount of exhibitionism, Aries tends to be a more experimental Sign, participating in dominance and submission and sometimes orgies. Libra finds straightforward sex more satisfying. It is a matter of degree. Libra enjoys talking about sex, eroticism more than pornography. Aries is quite comfortable getting down and dirty. Even in terms of sexual positions they have different preferences. Aries wants to be on top, Libra prefers doggie style and sixty-nine.

Libra loves luxury and wants to be treated well, wined and dined. Perhaps it's extreme to call Aries a cheapskate, but that's how Libra feels. For Aries, the perfect end of an evening is a roll in the hay. That's a far cry from a romantic picnic near the Golden Gate Bridge or a cappuccino in Provincetown.

When there's a decision to be made, Libra wants to explore all the avenues. Aries makes choices sooner than Libra can possibly look at those options. When Aries tells Libra "this is what I want to do," Libra has a thousand questions. Aries gets annoyed constantly explaining his rationale. In all, sex may be the best part of this relationship.

SUMMARY

Libra is attracted to that upbeat, youthful Aries attitude, which is true regardless of his age. Aries is drawn to Libra's unmistakably gentle, kind nature. They talk. Libra is attentive. Aries is exciting. The physical attraction is powerful. They get into the bedroom quickly. Aries is all about action and lust while Libra wants romance. Aries wants to hear "You are the best lover I ever had," even if he isn't. Libra wants to be praised for his looks, his body, his goodness as a person. If each waits for the other to stroke his ego, both will have decidedly hurt feelings.

Aries ~ Scorpio
The Ram and the Scorpion ~ fatal attraction

Aries is by nature uncomplicated, falling in love at first sight and wanting to go straight home to bed. Scorpio is a sign of great mystery. Initially Scorpio finds the directness, the "what you see is what you get" quality of Aries appealing, as well as puzzling, and goes looking for underlying innuendoes. Aries does not understand the depths of Scorpio, simply because Scorpio hides so much and Aries doesn't. Aries is a good-hearted, loyal, loving person, but Scorpio does not necessarily bring out the best in the Ram, and because Aries is so flirtatious, he brings out the worst of the Scorpion's jealous streak.

Aries, who is both vain and insecure, needs to be praised. Scorpio does little to ease this basic vulnerability. Competitive Aries wants to be the best. He likes to hear, "You're the best sex I've ever had." Scorpio, on the other hand, never wants to hear those words. Scorpio knows full well that Aries has had other lovers. Scorpio just does not want to be confronted with that fact.

In the bedroom, both Signs enjoy anal sex with Scorpio usually being the top. Scorpio enjoys ménage à trois, which is apt to make Aries insecure. Aries prefers the excitement of group sex in the anonymous setting of an orgy.

Scorpio wants to prove his sexual prowess and Aries is equally passionate. Each strives to impress the other. For sex, this is a great combination. For long-term relationships, it's not. Lust, yes. Love, no.

SUMMARY

The Ram is intensely drawn to passionate Scorpio. This is the fiery planet Mars meeting his sexual match. It's dynamic, instant, and fabulous sex, but both Scorpio and Aries are controlling signs so in the relationship one party has to be willing to concede. Aries is often in a hurry, absentminded about the impact or effect he is having on his partner. Scorpio may not say anything, but he is a highly emotional man and his feelings will be quite hurt. The sex may be fabulous, the friendship wonderful, but it isn't likely that these two men will form a lasting relationship.

Aries ~ **Sagittarius**
Ram and Archer ~ the arrow finds its mark

An enviable couple. These two Fire Signs make a fine relationship in bed and out. They share common interests from hiking and camping to gambling. They're both social beings who enjoy traveling, entertaining, and going out often. Aries enjoys playing the field, flirting, being with several lovers before settling down. Once committed, Aries is a steadfast partner and loyal friend. Likewise with Sagittarius, accepting grown-up responsibilities may be avoided as long as possible, but when accepted, Sagittarius is reliable, a hard worker, and a constant friend and lover.

Both Aries and Sagittarius are outgoing, Aries is more flamboyant than Sagittarius. Though Aries gives the impression of self-confidence, Sagittarius is actually more self-assured. Aries is a bit of a hot-head. Most of the time, Sagittarius is quite mellow and laid back, but you don't want to make The Archer angry. That temper may be rarely seen, but it's a force to deal with and, when released, it comes out in a torrent of very cutting remarks. Aries is easily wounded.

In their sexual life, Aries is more experimental, but finds Sagittarius a willing partner. Both get turned on by having sex in public places, especially in a forest or park, as long as there is real risk of being seen. Both signs enjoy anal sex with Aries assuming the role of top.

In the initial stages of a relationship, Sagittarius will let Aries run the show. Over time, in a fairly subtle way, Sagittarius will take over. If Aries resists, Sagittarius will be more forceful.

SUMMARY

The attraction is mutual and powerful. Sex is likely to begin almost at once as both Signs want to have sex on the first encounter. In bed, the well-endowed Sagittarius wants his penis praised. Aries wants to be told he's the best sex Sagittarius has ever had. Aries is used to taking charge, Sagittarius is not about to let that go on for long. Regarding who's in control here, some conflict is inevitable, but ultimately Aries will need to concede and Sagittarius will be gracious. As a couple, these two will have energy, charm, and magnetism enough to cause envy among other men.

Aries ~ Capricorn
The Ram and the Goat ~ conflicting species

This is something of a business deal in that with mutual effort each gets a substantial reward. Aries brings excitement to this relationship. Capricorn brings stability. But this is not an easy pairing.

Both Signs have some tendency to be flirtatious as well as at least a little jealous. The Ram, rued by the planet Mars, will let that Martian anger out. The Goat may withdraw in stony silence. In addition, Capricorn is so intent upon achieving and accomplishing in life that he may not put enough attention into the relationship. The Ram left too much to his own devises is apt to roam afield.

Aries recognizes the need for a partner who balances his impulsive nature. Capricorn does that. Capricorn is intrigued by the vitality of Aries and by the wonderful ability Aries has to be open to new things, without prejudging. Capricorn has an opinion about almost everything. With a prodigious memory, when confronting something new, the Goat puts it into a category with previous experiences. Aries approaches new things simply and openly.

In bed, though Aries is somewhat experimental, his preferences range from kissing to oral sex and intercourse. Many Capricorns want to experiment with a wider range of sexual behaviors that may go from light bondage into sado-masochism. The Goat must go slowly to initiate Aries, and Aries must be open-minded if sex is to remain vital. Can this relationship last, yes. Will it? That depends wholly on how much effort each brings to it.

SUMMARY

Capricorn can be straightforward to the point of bluntness, hurtful to Aries. Aries can be such a little boy, seeing life through his own somewhat naive perspective, whereas Capricorn gleans experience from many sources and develops a broader, perhaps older, outlook. It will always fall to Capricorn, therefore, to adjust and make allowances for Aries. Capricorn loves Aries vitality in bed, but he may find it hard to keep up with his pace. Capricorn may be more interested in anal activities whereas Aries is primarily oral. This relationship, though difficult, has its best chance if Capricorn is several years older than Aries.

Aries ~ Aquarius
The Ram and the Water Bearer ~ a challenge

Aquarius is enthusiastic about ideas. Aries is enthusiastic about life. As friends, business partners, or co-workers, they really hit it off. Sex is the only problem area. If it can be handled, these two will have a very successful, long-lasting relationship. Aquarius is a good intellectual lover, sometimes not a good physical lover. Aquarius knows what to do and can talk a partner to the edge of ecstasy, but there's often little real passion behind the performance.

Aries is like a first-grade school child, impulsive, impatient, and assertive. Aries lets a partner know what is desired and the Ram expects a mate to come through. Even in matters sexual, Aries will be impatient if those needs aren't being met. The Ram tries very hard to satisfy a partner, sometimes performing acts he doesn't enjoy all that much. Aries expects that kind of consideration in return.

Aquarius is like an eleventh grader, grown up, well mannered. Aquarius knows you don't always get what you want right now, that you have to be patient. Aries isn't patient. Aquarius is thoughtful and gifted at using words, conveying hopes and wishes. But the Water Bearer may seem somewhat aloof and detached while the Ram is entirely within the moment. Words excite Aquarius. Kissing and actions turn on Aries. Phone sex was probably invented by an Aquarian. After all, sex begins in the brain. Aries wants the real thing or nothing at all. It's actions, not words, that get the Ram turned on.

SUMMARY

If these two begin a sexual relationship quickly, they'll probably never have more than casual sex. Sex alone won't ignite burning desire for a lasting relationship. For Aquarius, the primary sex organ is his brain. For Aries it's firmly between his legs. These two can be great friends. With that foundation, they may find a way to create a satisfying sex life through ideas and communication. To turn on Aquarius, Aries might talk dirty over dinner, as foreplay is verbal. For Aquarius to turn on Aries, he must praise him repeatedly, "My what a good boy you are."

Aries ~ **Pisces**
The Ram and the Fish ~ an odd couple

Pisces, the twelfth Sign of the zodiac, "The Dustbin," collects some qualities of all previous signs. Pisces is rather like an onion, a sweet one of course, with layer upon layer. Aries is the first Sign of the zodiac. Pretty much what you see is what you get. Aries doesn't feel the need for subterfuge or diplomacy. Aries calls it like it is.

Pisceans seem able to get others to do their bidding so subtly, their artful manipulation goes unnoticed. Without aggression and effortlessly, Pisces prevails. Is it hypnosis? One thing's for sure, it's a far cry from Aries's no-holds-barred, direct, forthright approach. Pisces is the most sensitive zodiac Sign, while Aries can be pretty blunt.

Given these fundamental differences, these two often wind up in an on-again, off-again relationship. It will not be easy for them to stay together, and yet the effort can be well worth it. Aries is tough but also loyal and steadfast. Pisces cherishes those very qualities.

Initially this relationship is great in bed. Pisces sees Aries as wonderfully strong, a decided turn-on, as Pisces loves enduring sex. Later on, when Pisces discovers that Aries is still very much a child, the intensity dies out. Pisces loves sex to be like a screenplay. Aries doesn't want to go through all the romance, the lighting of candles, and incense, things that Pisces loves. Aries wants to get right to the main event. Pisces wants to enjoy seduction and setting the stage.

SUMMARY

Mature Pisces enjoys Aries's vitality and naïve approach to life, but if Pisces expects Aries to grow up and act his age, he's in for a rude awakening. For all that Aries appears independent, he needs someone to rely on. A strange inversion—Aries appears powerful while Pisces appears vulnerable. At the core, the reverse is more accurate. Pisces must be the dominant male, while Aries acts the part, for this relationship to work. In bed, Pisces will find that Aries isn't going to reach very far to accommodate him, and that he, Pisces, will have to take it or leave it.

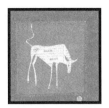

Taurus ~ Taurus
Two Bulls together ~ let's get physical

Frequently when two like Signs get together, there is competition, a sense of "who's in charge here." That's not the case with two Taurans. They love the same things: good food, a warm environment, and lengthy passionate sex. They're patient, kind, slow to anger, and loyal. They're romantic, and neither seeks to dominate the other. Even when it comes to their negative traits, each knows how to back off from the other rather than make a bad scene worse.

Taurus needs to be told "I love you," and Taurus accommodates. When one Bull is in a foul mood, the second knows not to press the issue. One needs a hug and the other complies. Above all else, Taurus needs stability and security and on an emotional level he finds it with a Taurus partner.

Sex is long, romantic, sensual, satisfying. It feels as though the whole world has stopped. They really enjoy each other, but they can go broke putting too much time into the physical side of life. In bed it's great, but some time they have to get up, go out, and earn their daily bread.

The sex life is fundamentally conservative, sticking to lots of kissing, touching, massaging, and anal sex. As a result, sex could become routine, in spite of each partner's regard for the other. In fantasy life, the sex is far more adventuresome. Exploring some of that side of sexuality, with an occasional can of whipped cream, introducing a sex toy, or wearing an unexpected costume, will add a certain spark.

SUMMARY

This is a thoroughly satisfying relationship in bed, in business, and in friendship. Both are practical, down to earth, and stable. They love creature comforts, including overstuffed armchairs, tons of pillows on the bed, a cozy fire on the hearth, and a pantry well stocked with food. They love talking with each other. They will enjoy cooking together and then eating their meals in the kitchen, in the den, or in the bedroom off fine china, paper plates, or bare skin. Equally matched in lovemaking approaches and preferences, routine never becomes boring. After all, if it ain't broke, why fix it?

Taurus ~ **Gemini**
The Twins and the Bull ~ friends and lovers

On the friendship side, these two Signs get along very well. Each has attributes the other needs. Gemini, as the Sign of experimentation, brings liveliness and versatility. Gemini introduces Taurus to a broad range of experiences. Taurus, as the Sign of stability and security, provides grounding and practicality. While Gemini's attention might wander, Taurus is ever steadfast and loyal. These factors account for the longevity of so many Gemini/Taurus relationships.

In the bedroom, there are substantial differences in style and pleasure. Taurus doesn't mind setting a date for sex. Gemini wants spontaneity. Taurus is content with about a half hour for lovemaking, Gemini might want more time. Variety doesn't necessarily turn on Taurus. Gemini wants to experiment. Taurus, the most physical sign in the zodiac, just loves sex. He wants to be touched, kissed, licked, and sucked and is thoroughly satisfied with repetitive foreplay. That would prove monotonous for Gemini.

The most difficult area for these two is their approach to problem-solving. Gemini does multiple tasks at once, having a remarkable ability to focus on that one thing on which he is currently involved, undistracted by all the other piles of unfinished business. Taurus does one thing and becomes unnerved by Gemini's seeming chaos. When worried, Gemini withdraws from the stress-producing situation and simply redirects focus to one of those myriad other endeavors. When Taurus is worried, there can be no other involvement. Taurus is relentless.

Still, Taurus's patience and Gemini's good nature combine to help these two maintain a loving connection.

SUMMARY

Taurus is a devoted mate, stable, and perhaps a tad boring, not necessarily to everyone, but he can be for a Gemini, who moves and thinks quickly and is into so many things simultaneously. When Gemini comes to appreciate these wonderful Taurus traits, he may find that "boring" is replaced by "committed." Gemini's curiosity about the world, his interest in politics, restaurants, even local gossip, all add breath and excitement to the Bull's life. Sex will be more gratifying if Gemini demonstrates more affection. He doesn't give random hugs or touch his partner often. Taurus wants those signs of his partner's affection.

Taurus ~ **Cancer**
The Bull and the Crab ~ contented combo

Picture two kids playing in the mud, having a wonderful time, and you've got an image of Taurus with Cancer. This can be one of the most successful relationships in the zodiac.

Both love their home, wanting to create an environment that is welcoming. They enjoy working in their gardens and preparing food for friends and family. Planning and cooking a meal together is a sexual experience. They are affectionate and openly loving and nurturing to each other. They both have patient and tenacious natures. Even in their lesser traits each provides balance for the other. Cancer is a worrier. Taurus is reassuring. Taurus frets about money. Cancer is confident about helping to provide it.

When Cancer is upset he wants to talk. Taurus is a great listener. When Taurus is upset and ready to talk, Cancer not only makes a wonderful listener, but also has a real knack for drawing Taurus out. Cancer is a sucker for a sob story, wanting to kiss it and make it better, and Taurus, strong and independent in some regards, appreciates a loving shoulder to lean on.

In the sexual arena they both enjoy fairly lengthy foreplay, touching, and deep kissing, but then they diverge. Taurus is primarily satisfied with a mainstream range of sex, including oral and anal sex. Cancer is quite open to a greater range of expression. For this couple's sex life to remain satisfying, Cancer must move slowly and Taurus must be willing to expand his sexual behaviors.

SUMMARY

Here is a relationship likely to last through the ages with an enviable depth of caring and commitment. Both men strive to avoid confrontation, are sensitive and respectful of each other's feelings. Their depth of friendship is another help in those difficult times that all relationships encounter. It is unlikely that there will be any problems in the bedroom as long as each partner is willing to accommodate the other's desires. The only real area of potential conflict, if you want to call it that, is that Cancer loves to make love in the woods while Taurus prefers plush pillows to pine needles.

Taurus ~ **Leo**
The Bull and the Lion ~ incompatible species

Taurus and Leo, both fixed Signs, respect each other. Taurus represents practicality and tenacity. Leo represents creativity, the willingness to take chances. In business and friendship, these qualities serve as checks and balances for each other. In love relationships, however, there are problems.

Leo is prone to snap judgments. Taurus takes a long time making decisions. Leo may misinterpret this slowness of pace as indecisiveness. Wrong call. If Leo then tries to rush Taurus, Taurus will prove how well he deserves to be called bullheaded. Even in the way they work out their personal concerns, these two are different. Leo doesn't worry, resolving problems quickly. Taurus takes time going over and over issues, which Leo finds tedious.

While both are flirtatious, Leo's outgoing, flamboyant nature triggers Taurus's insecurity. In addition, though both Signs are highly passionate, they have very different approaches and behaviors sexually. Leo wants variety, spontaneity, exploration, and a sense of urgency to feed passion. Leo wants play in the sexual act.

For Taurus, passion is more about length, duration of the sex act, and Taurus doesn't do much exploring other than to participate in a ménage à trois, which is not often to Leo's liking. In addition, Taurus is content with the conventional range of sex, hand holding, deep kissing, fondling, mutual masturbation, oral and anal sex. Leo wants something more unconventional and a greater sense of ecstasy. Without that, Leo gets bored.

Taurus needs stability and security. Leo is extravagant. Taurus is straightforward and conservative. Leo is flamboyant, even outrageous. Initially exciting, long-term, they are at odds with each other.

SUMMARY

Leo optimism and willingness to fly by the seat of his pants as well as his flirtatiousness are unsettling to the Bull. The Lion has supreme confidence in himself but nonetheless he thrives on praise. Perhaps it's because he wants to be reassured that his greatness is being properly recognized. Most of the time Taurus is willing to comply. But Taurus is pretty competent in his own right, and this ongoing need of Leo's, to have his mane stroked, can get tedious. It would be better to stroke elsewhere.

Taurus ~ **Virgo**
The Bull and the Virgin ~ potent potential

These two Earth Signs, practical, straightforward, and caring, make for a great combination in all regards—friendship, business, and love. While Taurus has great need for security and stability, Virgo's methodical, detail-oriented qualities are reassuring. Virgo, which makes a great friend, ready to help out, not looking for a pat on the back, is deeply appreciative of the loyalty and steadfastness of Taurus.

Taurus and Virgo inherently trust each other and generally appreciate similar activities, centered on their home, food, and the pleasure of a close circle of intimate friends. They derive great comfort out of togetherness, whether tending their garden or preparing dinners. They aren't likely to argue often and get over it fairly quickly when they do.

Problems in this relationship are few. They may arise when Taurus is self-indulgent or lazy and when Virgo is nit-picking or faultfinding. Since Virgo works so hard at all aspects of life, he feels taken advantage of when a partner doesn't make an equal effort. Taurus is easily wounded by criticism.

Sexually, highly physical Taurus, loving to lick, suck, and kiss, is gratified by Virgo's responsive hands caressing and fondling Taurus. If there ever are any problems in the bedroom, they come from the fact that Taurus is content with traditional sexual expression while Virgo may want to experience a far greater range of behaviors. If Virgo goes slowly, Taurus will gradually comply and respond enthusiastically. If rushed, Taurus will prove itself worthy of its symbol, the Bull.

SUMMARY

The initial heat may yield to a marked degree of surprise on the part of Taurus. How could it possibly be that Virgo is called "the Virgin?" Many Virgo men will try virtually anything, anytime, and maybe even anywhere. From bondage to sex toys, role playing to piercings, Virgo is often front and center. The foundation of trust between these signs is likely to help Taurus overcome, what might be, some conservative constraints. Where Taurus longs for a committed partner he's likely to find that in Virgo. Here are two Signs ready to be steady, consistent, committed, and loving.

Taurus ~ **Libra**
The Bull and the Scales ~ almost on the balance point

Thrilling, passionate, and romantic, both Signs are ruled by Venus, the planet of love and luxury. Taurus is an Earth Sign, highly physical, loves to touch, and uses body language to express sexual needs and wants. Libra is an Air Sign, a Sign of communication, turned on verbally and communicates sexual wants more with words than body language.

Both Signs enjoy taking their time, up to an hour, sometimes more, for each sexual encounter, and find quickies either not enjoyable or only fun on occasion. Food is a turn-on. For Taurus, sharing food is enough to turn thoughts to sex. For Libra it can be fun to incorporate food with sex. In the sex act itself, Taurus loves the physicality, all the touching, while Libra loves the romance, the wine, music, and candlelight.

There are important differences. Libra is an independent Sign, and while Taurus is a strong personality, the Sign has a dependent streak. The result is Taurus may seem clinging or controlling to Libra, whereas, Libra's self-contained behavior triggers insecurities in Taurus. Libra is ever the romantic, sentimental, enjoying small tokens of love. Taurus is far more practical and, when it comes to receiving gifts, would prefer that a lover would save up and buy something of consequence rather than wasting money on trivial trinkets.

This is not an easy twosome, though a lifelong relationship is possible. Taurus must work at being a more interesting conversationalist, and Libra must focus more attention on the sex act itself.

SUMMARY

They make great business partners or friends as they share many interests from dog shows to antiquing. They care about the home environment and enjoy beautiful things. They may be artistic or at least appreciate the arts. But in an intimate relationship, they aren't well matched. Libra is more social and wants to party. Taurus wants to stay home. Between the sheets, Taurus wants a lot of touching and exploring. Libra wants to get to the point. Taurus wants a seven-course meal; he is the dessert. Libra enjoys sex before doing something else, after something else, but never instead of something else.

Taurus ~ **Scorpio**
The Bull and the Scorpion ~ opposites attract and repel

Taurus and Scorpio are opposite signs and opposites do attract, but that attraction may only work for the short term. Taurus is quite direct, often blunt. Scorpio is guarded in speech. When Taurus is upset and ready to talk, Taurus will talk a blue streak. Secretive Scorpio, always afraid of saying too much, afraid of revealing too much, may find that behavior disarmingly attractive, for a while. Later, Scorpio is apt to become bored with Taurus's long tirades. Another problem is that Taurus's energy level is so different from Scorpio's. Scorpio is driven. Taurus has a lazy streak.

On the positive side, Taurus finds Scorpio receptive and understanding. Taurus wants protecting and Scorpio gladly complies. Regarding sex, Taurus is the most physical Sign in the zodiac, loves to touch and be touched. Taurus is extremely sensual in all regards, luxuriating in warmth whether in front of the fireplace or at the beach in sunny climes. Taurus loves music. Taurus is very oral and food is a turn-on. Scorpio, with its highly sexy nature, matches the passion of Taurus.

Taurus makes a great life partner, extremely loyal, never tolerating anyone speaking ill of his or her lover. Where Scorpio wants a profound relationship, yearns for a soul mate, Taurus can provide gratification. The problems come in when Taurus gets possessive. Scorpio's need for freedom causes Taurus's insecurity. Taurus hates change and Scorpio is forever changing things. Can this relationship work? Yes. Will it? All depends upon how these two choose to behave.

SUMMARY

The sex is great in bed, in a car, or in a secluded grove. Scorpio will try most anything and Taurus is accommodating, from oil slathered on a plastic sheet to creative uses of hot dog buns and whipped cream. Where Scorpio wants commitment, Taurus provides loyalty. Scorpio will want to be the dominant partner, and as long as he's a good provider, Taurus will comply. Taurus has to beware of spending more rapidly than Scorpio earns. Generally Taurus is a great cook, and where Scorpio may not attend overly well to his diet, Taurus will make sure that he does.

Taurus ~ **Sagittarius**
The Bull and the Archer ~ curious balance

This is a potentially fantastic relationship, surprisingly because they have many fundamental differences. Taurus craves stability and security. Sagittarius is a risk taker. Taurus is a bit of a coach potato. Sagittarius says, "Don't fence me in." Taurus is sensitive and easily wounded. Sagittarius tends to shoot from the hip. Taurus prefers a life that centers on home entertaining and cookouts in the back yard. Sagittarius is an active Sign, enjoying travel, sports, and gambling. Taurus is a planner and Sagittarius is spontaneous.

What Taurus and Sagittarius have in common, helping to overcome these disparities, is that they both love food and enjoy doing a variety of things together, as long as it is not too often for Taurus or too repetitive for Sagittarius. Taurus is ruled by the planet Venus, representing sensual pleasures, while Sagittarius is ruled by Jupiter, the planet that rules extravagance and expansion. In a curious way, the stable, earth-bound Taurus energy can prove comforting to the wanderlust nature of Sagittarius, and the expansiveness and desire for broad horizons of Sagittarius helps shake Taurus loose.

The sex is wonderful. Taurus likes it long and slow and Sagittarius has great endurance, like the Eveready bunny, going and going and going. Sagittarius enjoys several experimental behaviors, including dominance and submission, spanking, and bondage. Taurus tends to be rather mainstream in sexual expression but he is willing to explore. Sagittarius may be into sex toys. That's not a turn-on for Taurus. Both Signs like to incorporate food with sex.

SUMMARY

The number one problem here may be over money. Sagittarius is seldom concerned about cash coming in. Taurus needs to know that his partner's share of the bills will be paid. If the Bull thinks his partner is letting things slide, he'll take on more of the responsibility for a while then finally blow his top. On the plus side, life's little problems seldom bother the Archer and this proves reassuring to his partner. But for Taurus to feel truly secure in the relationship, Sagittarius needs to be more sensitive. For Sagittarius to know where he stands, Taurus needs to speak up rather than let hurts fester and grow.

Taurus ~ Capricorn
The Bull and the Goat ~ mutual admiration

This is a fine relationship, a mutual admiration society. They work through their infrequent disagreements with little stress. Taurus and Capricorn are Earth Signs with equally strong libidos and can expect to have a lasting and enjoyable sex life. It isn't necessarily fireworks, but it is a slow and steady burn.

Taurans and most Capricorns are mainstream sexually, very into touch and kissing. They love to take their time in each sexual encounter, lingering over foreplay. Both want about thirty minutes to an hour for sex, half that for foreplay and love to achieve orgasm at the same time.

Some Capricorns are into the BDSM lifestyle . . . wanting to explore the range of sexual practices of bondage, dominance and submission, and sadomasochism. The Goat may be able to coax the Bull into role-playing and bondage but not likely into accepting pain as part of the pleasure. If Taurus adopts the dominant role and Capricorn the submissive, this may work out better.

Neither Taurus nor Capricorn will be hurried. With Taurus, if one tries to get Taurus to make a decision quickly, the Bull will almost always say "no." They do not want to be trapped into an unhappy situation by too hastily saying "yes." Capricorn is a patient Sign, not likely to hurry Taurus. Taurus is not disturbed when Capricorn, who prefers to think things through without discussion, shares a decision only after having made it alone. In any kind of relationship, sexual or business, these two have most everything going for them.

SUMMARY

Some couples have trouble communicating. Not these two. Their greatest strength is a kind of mutual directness in speech and action. Problems between them are few but one is significant. Taurus can be quite emotional and Capricorn may not know how to handle him. The solution is simple. An upset Bull needs two things. He needs to be hugged and he needs to be fed. Once Taurus relaxes over dinner or a cup of coffee, he opens up, gets talking and the problem is en route to being solved. Conversely when the Goat has a nagging concern, he finds Taurus a remarkably good listener.

Taurus ~ **Aquarius**
The Bull and the Water Bearer ~ no common ground

Just think of these two symbols: the cool, calm Water Bearer versus the mighty and dangerous Bull. That's what putting these two Signs together into a love relationship amounts to. There's no common ground.

Initially Taurus, who can be a bit reticent, is attracted by the Aquarian's ability to "work the crowd." Aquarius is everybody's buddy, having an extraordinary ability to fit in. The Water Bearer does the talking and finds a great listener in the Bull. As a friendship it's just fine. In intimate relationships, the problems are many.

Their pace and timing in life is at odds with each other. Together they create imbalance. Taurus moves slowly and hates to be rushed. Aquarius is a quick thinker and is off and running long before Taurus has digested the situation.

The diplomat of the zodiac, Aquarius is an Air Sign. In a crisis this is the person who knows how to stay focused on a rational, thinking plane, whereas Taurus, the Earth Sign, gets right to the physical. He wants to know what needs to be done, fixed, replaced, or repaired. Aquarius is thinking far ahead and expanding the perspective. They annoy each other. Aquarius says, "It's important to look at the big picture." Taurus says, "There's too much to do right here."

Sex is a similar problem. Aquarius wants to talk about sex. Taurus wants to just do it. They aren't in sync and thus satisfying the other becomes more pain than pleasure. Over time, Taurus is dissatisfied; Aquarius is bored.

SUMMARY

Taurus is comfortable with intimacy, one to one and with a small circle of friends. Aquarius may be ill at ease in these settings. Taurus is usually close to his relatives. Aquarius not necessarily so. Sexually, those Taurans and Aquarians whose range of behaviors is broadest, have the greatest chance to satisfy each other in the bedroom, sharing an interest in such things as using food, dildoes, and participating in water sports. Taurus is highly physical and into touching and cuddling, usually content with the tried and true repertoire. Most Aquarians seek variety of sensation through experimenting. Not a happy pair.

Taurus ~ **Pisces**
The Bull and the Fish ~ soul mates in paradise

From the bedroom to the boardroom these two relate well. Both are sensitive, caring, and loyal Signs. Taurus provides practicality and Pisces provides intuition.

Highly emotional Pisces opens the feeling side of Taurus. Taurus provides quiet strength to Pisces who needs time to retreat and meditate. While some Sun Signs might be uncomfortable with these silent periods, Taurus is completely at ease with them.

Taurus is prone to worry about stability and security, about financial welfare. Pisces is a calming and confident influence, believing in their ability as a couple to resolve any problems.

Although there are very few problems for these two, one might arise from the Bull's tendency to be abrupt, which can trigger Pisces defensiveness. Another comes from the Pisces trait to avoid discord by agreeing to go along a certain course, even when that's not the Fish's opinion, and then going right back to doing whatever he was doing before.

Taurus is ruled by Venus, the planet of physical love. Pisces is ruled by Neptune, the planet of spiritual love. These two share a love affair that plays on both levels, making the relationship a true soul mate connection. Sex is instinctively right. Taurus is a mainstream lover but quite vocal, and Pisces being a romantic, very invested in bringing pleasure to a partner, is gratified to hear sounds of ecstasy. Pisces has great endurance. Taurus loves long, slow sex. Nobody needs to coach this happy couple, and the relationship can be fulfilling lifelong.

SUMMARY

Neither is the macho, aggressive type. Neither is perceived as decisive, take charge. Yet both are strong, quiet, and capable of considerable accomplishments. They provide each other the kind of backup and support that bring out the best in each. Where Pisces may seem insecure or too much the dreamer, Taurus grounds him, gives him direction. Where Taurus may be too locked into practicality, Pisces opens his eyes to spirituality and mysteries. This is a happy pair in public and private, with and without clothes on. In fact in the bedroom, each feels secure enough to let down all guards and relish the physicality.

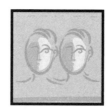

Gemini ~ Gemini
Two Twins together ~ complement or chaos?

Just imagine one hundred piles of unfinished business belonging to Gemini #1 and one hundred piles of unfinished business belonging to Gemini #2. And there you have it, life for two Geminis together, mutual chaos, and nobody cares. Of course, somebody's got to go to the market, take out the trash, and pay the bills. One thing's for sure; these two better maintain separate checking accounts.

They can talk with each other for hours, never running out of things to say. They love exploring a wide spectrum of life together. In the beginning, it's exciting, as Gemini feels unique among people, and here he encounters a mirror image. But in fact, too much similarity is a problem. They get into power struggles and both are apt to be dealing simultaneously with parallel difficulties.

In the bedroom, at first it's stimulating as each tries to impress the other with style and variety. But something is missing, the spark of a Fire Sign or the endurance of Earth. Over time, there just isn't enough variety and both become bored.

The tendency to be inconstant or shallow may also be exaggerated when two Geminis team up. In addition, Gemini is flirtatious and can be jealous, and they trigger insecurities in each other. In time, each Gemini feels a longing for a partner who provides a stimulus or presents a feeling of stability, of being balanced or grounded. All these behaviors outside the bedroom undermine the relationship and everything backfires on them. It is hardly likely to work.

SUMMARY

Shouldn't it be satisfying to be with an exciting partner who never runs out of things to say, who is a perfect match intellectually and shares a desire to constantly learn new things? Sounds right, but there are problems. Gemini is not very likely to make a long-term commitment. He is monogamous to the extent that the relationship lasts. That might be a few weeks or a few months. If each can overlook the other's flirtations, what exists is a wonderful friendship with mutual interests and goals, and a relationship that can be highly gratifying, at least for a while.

Gemini ~ Cancer
The Twins and the Crab ~ sex: sure fire, relationship: doubtful

Here we have two Sun Signs about as alike as night and day, and yet between the sheets it's a great sexual combination. Both Sun Signs range from experimental to very open in their sexual behaviors. Gemini lights Cancer's emotional fires, perhaps too much so. Cancer believes that Gemini shares the same feelings, but Gemini doesn't.

Cancer comes from a feeling core, while Gemini comes from a more intellectual place. In other words, Cancer buys into the game and the sexual role-playing, wholeheartedly with emotion and passion. Sex and love become wrapped up and synonymous. Gemini on the other hand, manages to occupy the roles of experimenter and observer simultaneously, enjoying sex, loving sex, but seeing it as apart from or other than love. While Cancer gives himself over with full abandon, Gemini retains a certain emotional distance. For Cancer, this complexity can create a kind of emotion maelstrom that may be too much to sustain.

Aside from the sex, personality trait by personality trait, these two have little in common. Gemini is restless and won't allow anyone to pin him down while Cancer is possessive. Cancer clings. Gemini tries to gain distance. Cancer grows insecure and tries to hold on harder. Cancer feels deeply whereas Gemini shies away from emotion. Gemini is a nervous sign and Cancer worries. Each sets off the other. They may love each other all the while driving each other to distraction. On a scale of 1 to 10, sex scores 10. Relationship only 4.

SUMMARY

The best long-term prognosis for this couple is when Gemini is older than Cancer by seven years or more. Cancer is loving, devoted, steadfast, but also moody, emotional, and clingy. The relationship is difficult until Gemini is mature enough to appreciate those wonderful positive qualities without being turned off by the negative ones. However, if Gemini is considerably younger than his Cancer lover, the Cancer in question needs to overlook Gemini's flirtatious nature. Sex is the best part of their relationship. Gemini's approach is more intellectual than sensual, while Cancer is passionately involved in performance. Sexually they inspire each other.

Gemini ~ Leo
The Twins and the Lion ~ potential paradise

They love to talk, dance, and travel. They truly complement each other. Gemini loves to experiment and Leo loves to explore. Between the sheets this is a great combination. The one real obstacle to long-term bliss for this couple is that Gemini's flirtatiousness makes Leo intensely jealous. Leo, so full of himself, won't put up with that. Gemini must curb the "friendly" act or Leo will take off, and a potential lifelong relationship will dissolve.

What Fire Sign Leo brings to Gemini is a spark of vitality, and Air Sign Gemini keeps the experience going. Leo might be a bit single-minded in approaching sex, passionate but set in specific ways or might rush too quickly to climax. Gemini provides a balance. Gemini wants to talk things through, "Why are you doing that? What's that all about?" For Leo, sex is always hot and heavy. Gemini tempers things, which proves very satisfactory to Leo.

Leo likes being praised, adored in fact. Gemini, attention elsewhere, may forget to lavish compliments. Leo, being outrageously self-confident, will overlook this Gemini lapse most of the time. But for these two to be truly happy, Gemini needs to remember that the Lion loves to have his mane stroked and responds with lavish generosity when it is.

For Gemini, the biggest problem with Leo is that Leo is always right. In a disagreement, therefore, Gemini must be wrong. Clearly Leo needs to give Gemini more credit for his wonderful intellect and ability to solve problems.

SUMMARY

The Leo man enters a room with an aura of self-confidence that turns all heads. He doesn't need to flirt to draw attention to himself. Gemini works the crowd, flitting from group to group, a witty word and a ready laugh. These two are, unquestionably, a natural pair, as long as Gemini doesn't resent the amount of attention that Leo commands and Leo doesn't mind the flirtatiousness of his Gemini lover. Should jealousy arise between these two, it's all over. One problem, Leo is extravagant and money concerns will trigger Gemini's nervousness. Here Leo's light-hearted reassurances won't work. Budgeting will.

Gemini ~ Virgo
The Twins and the Virgin ~ crazy-making situation

Somewhere in the vast expanse of Mother Earth there are some happy Gemini/Virgo couples, but they are rare. These two have so little in common. Earth Sign Virgo generally deadens the Air for Gemini, who gets bored with Virgo's systematic approach to all of life, including sexuality. Gemini, wanting to try something new, somewhere else, somehow differently, makes Virgo fundamentally uncomfortable.

In a curious way, Gemini and Virgo have something important in common, a sense of order. Virgo knows exactly where everything is. The Virgo environment is tightly organized. Even when Virgo has many possessions and lives in a small place, there is seldom any clutter. Gemini loves clutter but in the midst of chaos can find anything. This form of order is beyond Virgo's comprehension. They drive each other berserk.

There are two types in the Virgo Sun Sign: those who are mainstream in their sexuality and those who are open in their willingness to experiment. In bed, mainstream Virgo is wonderful with his hands, and there is a set pattern to his behavior. For Gemini that predictability undermines passion. Virgo longs for eroticism. Gemini wants raw sex. Virgo gets immersed in the act. Gemini remains something of an observer.

Sex for Gemini and the more experimental Virgo is more satisfying, at least briefly, because Gemini enjoys trying out variations of sexual behaviors and sex toys galore. But even here, Virgo is likely to slip into routine, boring Gemini and Gemini's desire for constant change is likely to unnerve Virgo.

SUMMARY

Virgo worries and Gemini gets nervous. Gemini needs someone to take his mind off his stress. Virgo needs someone to walk him through his worries. This incompatibility extends into the bedroom. Worried Virgo has little sex drive. He can't focus on anything until he has a handle on his problems. For Gemini, sex is the perfect cure for everything from the common cold to job-related stress. It distracts him and distraction is the best bromide for Gemini's edginess. As a friendship, this pairing may be wonderful. But as a love affair, it will be short-lived and as a commitment, unlikely.

Gemini ~ Libra
The Twins and the Scales ~ sensual seduction

The foundation of the Gemini/Libra relationship is their ability to communicate. They spend ten minutes having sex, then two hours discussing it. They could write the greatest romance novels together. Each tells the other, "I adore the feel of your hands on my skin. No one else has ever excited me so much." They look at each other lovingly, adoringly, and blissfully. This is truly a mutual admiration society. They are content with each other in the outside world and at home in bed.

Libra debates extensively between two possibilities, whereas Gemini tends to explore dozens of them. In a relationship, each is comfortable with the other's need to discuss multiple options. The only problem between these two verbally is that when Gemini gets upset, he is apt to say something that is quite cruel and cutting. Refined Libra rarely retaliates but always remembers.

Both Signs are affectionate by nature and rather easygoing. They will have a very active sex life that is both varied and fun, though it won't be overly passionate. Libra loves romance, while Gemini tends to get too quickly to the heart of the matter. If Libra brings variety into the bedroom, Gemini's curiosity will result in improved sex.

The one issue that could undermine their sex life would be money problems. Libra loves luxury. Gemini may be disorganized. If neither attends to the checkbook and financial problems ensue, Gemini grows nervous and Libra becomes irritable. Not the best energies to take into the bedroom.

SUMMARY

Sexual compatibility and ease discussing almost any subject on earth keep these two happy in and out of bed. The only problem area has to do with the practical realities of life. As long as these can be divided up fairly, Libra being responsible for the financial aspects and Gemini paying attention to the details, or vice-versa, all should go well. Neither partner seeks to dominate. In terms of who's in charge here, they alternate. Both Signs are dual by nature, meaning they both need considerable variety in their lives, new places to visit, people to meet, and things to explore.

Gemini ~ Scorpio
The Twins and the Scorpion ~ rarely the twain shall meet

Variety, including the use of external stimulation, X-rated videos, and sex toys, triggers Gemini's sexuality as well as Scorpio's. But primarily, Gemini is turned on by words while Scorpio is excited by emotion, feeling close. For a while, what they have in common is other interests, from travel to the arts, ideas about education and politics, helps these two out. Ultimately, the differences put a strain on the relationship. Scorpio is jealous. Gemini is flirtatious. Potential disaster.

They do virtually everything differently. Scorpio always takes the same street to get to a given, familiar destination. Gemini will find three alternate routes. They get into the car, Scorpio expects Gemini to turn right. Gemini turns left. This sounds like a minor thing, but cumulatively it's annoying, and in bed it turns Scorpio off. Scorpio wants a certain kind of foreplay. Gemini does something else. The result is less than a rip-roaring "O."

While Gemini does myriad things at once, Scorpio moves inexorably toward one objective. Scorpio grows impatient, as Gemini seems to leave everything dangling. Gemini just doesn't understand why Scorpio can't be more flexible. In addition, these two do not communicate well. Scorpio says something, Gemini's attention is elsewhere, and he doesn't hear Scorpio. When triggered emotionally, Gemini uses words hurtfully. Scorpio never forgets and the words leave scars.

A long-distance relationship can work well for these two. They'd have time apart to devote to their separate interests. When together, Gemini would then focus the attention, sexually and otherwise, that Scorpio requires.

SUMMARY

Gemini moves on from one interest to another and from one endeavor to another. Scorpio stays on one path. Gemini makes a game of finding new ways to do everyday things. Scorpio is disconcerted. Scorpio doesn't want to think about how to do mundane things. Let it become routine and Scorpio can move on to more important matters. For Gemini all things are a part of the game. Neither is right, merely different, but the differences undermine the comfort between them and ultimately destroy the sex as well. Add to that Gemini's flirtatiousness and Scorpio's jealousy, and you have an unhappy twosome.

Gemini ~ Sagittarius
The Twins and the Archer ~ opposites attract and repel

Gemini and Sagittarius are opposite signs, which is both stimulating and difficult. The relationship is a struggle, rather like climbing a mountain, but that's a turn-on for Gemini. Unfortunately their differences in temperament—Gemini has something of a detached quality, Sagittarius displays more fiery passion—result in terrible sexual timing. When Gemini wants to take time, Sagittarius wants a quickie. And yet they have many similarities in likes and dislikes. Both are sexually experimental, open to role-playing, bondage, and incorporating food with sex.

Neither Sign is possessive. Sagittarius is the laissez-faire Sign of the zodiac, "I won't tell you what to do, don't tell me what to do." Gemini too has a restless need to be unfettered. But in too many ways, they bring out the worst in each other. Sagittarius loves a good debate, even something of a verbal fight. Gemini finds this nerve-wracking. Sagittarius can cut loose with stinging barbs and is an inveterate tease. Gemini hates being teased and may retaliate with cruel words. They both have long memories and these exchanges build up resentment over time.

Gemini needs a variety of life experiences before settling down into one direction or with a life partner. Sagittarius struggles to find a balance between freedom and responsibility. Gemini is not ready for a committed relationship until the age of twenty-nine. Neither is Sagittarius, which is also known as the bachelor Sign of the zodiac. If these two take their time forming a committed relationship, there's more hope long-term.

SUMMARY

This relationship has its best chance if they come together in their thirties or if Sagittarius is around seven years older than Gemini. Sagittarius is the all-American stud, reputedly very well endowed. He loves young, smooth skin, and Gemini is remarkable for staying young looking well into middle age. Older Sagittarius is likely to have settled down, retreating from climbing mountains to reading travelogues. His broad interests enliven conversations with Gemini and Gemini's love of play and versatility in bed turn him on. They will be happiest as a couple if each is very involved in his own separate activities.

Gemini ~ Capricorn
The Twins and the Goat ~ success behind closed doors

This combination is surprisingly successful. Air Signs like Gemini and Earth Signs like Capricorn usually stifle each other, but these two create balance. Why does it work? Because Gemini needs to be grounded and Capricorn is very pragmatic. Geminis are quite scattered in many aspects of life and have a tendency to move from one thing to another without going far enough toward the heart of any matter. Capricorn starts on a path and is relentless in achieving his ambitions. Conversely, Capricorns can be too rooted to one spot. Gemini's multifaceted nature opens Capricorn to variety and to experiencing more of life. Gemini's youthful attitude helps lighten Capricorn up.

Gemini may not be materialistic but likes the opportunities that money brings. Hard-working Capricorn is generally quite successful. Perhaps he will contribute more to this twosome's budget. In return, Gemini's ongoing interest in learning new things, willingness to try new things, will keep Capricorn satisfied in the bedroom and out.

A good many Capricorns are experimental sexually, keeping sex interesting for Gemini. With Gemini's tendency to be at once observer and participant, the added stimulus of behaviors, such as bondage, dominance and submission, and using sex toys, keeps this Sign focused. With the more mainstream Capricorn, Gemini is the one who brings experimentation into their sex life.

This pair faces two problems. First, Gemini is flirtatious and Capricorn has enormous pride. If Gemini is too friendly in the wrong circumstances, Capricorn will be mortified. Second, conservative Capricorn's need for order can be inhibiting to Gemini.

SUMMARY

These two can have such fun together if Capricorn relaxes his guard and allows himself to be entertained by Gemini's youthful, playful demeanor. Capricorn takes life so seriously. He's so grown up. Even as a little boy he was more mature than the other children. Gemini still plays with his food when he's seventy. Even in bed, Gemini wants his toys and, of course, Capricorn gets quite a charge out of bondage and leather and those sexy policeman uniforms. When Gemini gets terribly nervous, Capricorn can turn on the vacuum cleaner to calm him right down.

Gemini ~ Aquarius
The Twins and the Water Bearer ~
if not lovers, always friends

Gemini charm meets Aquarian friendliness. These two Air Signs have a wonderful ability to communicate endlessly. Most people talk primarily about themselves. These two are curious about the world at large, certainly about their community, and perhaps, especially, about their neighbors. They make great friends as well as successful business partners. All that's needed is somebody to be practical enough to take care of the nitty-gritty details. Easier said than done.

Aquarius is wonderful at brainstorming and bringing up streams of exciting ideas but not at making the ideas into realities. Gemini may be overwhelmed by the vastness of the Aquarian's concepts and is apt to rule out ways of implementing them as fast as Aquarius contrives them.

Aquarius is most at ease in a crowd and knows everyone casually. Gemini may feel slighted because the Water Bearer is so busy with all these other people. "You do not pay enough attention to me, you are too busy with your friends."

There is a fundamental coolness in the nature of both Aquarius and Gemini. In love relationships each longs for intimacy and yet is uncomfortable with it. Their sex life can be rich and varied as they compensate for this inherent lack of passion with wide-ranging searches for sensation. Sound is always a stimulus. For Gemini that may be music. For both Signs that will include dirty talk, watching erotic movies, and occasionally pornography. This can be a lifelong, comfortable, and successful, if not overly passionate, relationship.

SUMMARY

These two have a wonderful time talking and sharing activities. Aquarius is a voyeur. Give him something to look at and he is a lot more fun to play with. So if Gemini brings on the sex toys, lovemaking with Aquarius improves dramatically. Outside the bedroom, the relationship is comfortable when events in life are moving smoothly. In tough times, neither is adequately comforting to the other. When Aquarius is distressed, Gemini's nervous response is unsettling. When Gemini is upset, the Aquarius's cool, calm and collected behavior may be perceived as unfeeling. These two make better friends than lovers.

Gemini ~ Pisces
The Twins and the Fish ~ for the drama, an audience

Their differences are significant. Pisces is turned on by the sense of touch, intense hugging, fondling, and also passionate kissing. Gemini's approach is as much intellectual, observing, as it is sensory. Pisces is carried away by emotion. Pisces has extraordinary endurance in the bedroom. Gemini enjoys lingering over sex only some of the time

And yet, there are strong connections. Pisces is a dual-natured Sign, sometimes vibrant and dynamic and other times moody and self-pitying. Gemini, also dual natured, generally easygoing, has periods when he can be very negative. Should that coincide with a self-pitying period for Pisces, the air will be heavy with thunderclouds.

In spite of these difficulties, this relationship has the potential to be fun and satisfying. For one thing, the flexibility of their natures helps this partnership flourish. From eating Indian food to Mexican cuisine, Thai to a pig roast, both Signs are willing to dip in. In the bedroom, Gemini wants to fool around with various toys. Pisces says, "The more the merrier." Pisces wants to approach sex as if it were a drama with Pisces as the leading victim. Gemini says, "Sure why not? I'll play."

If they enjoy making a game of sex, with one responsible for setting the stage on Monday, the other responsible for Thursday, all goes well. If Gemini falls into sexual routine, resisting romance, Pisces will turn off. Conversely, now and then Pisces must allow Gemini a quickie without any particular build-up so that Gemini can release some nervous tension.

SUMMARY

Gemini gets into a sexual habit. He touches this place, he sucks on that place, and he expects everything will be ready for the grand finale. While Pisces likes to be guided by his lover, routine turns him off. Here Pisces must take the initiative and instruct Gemini. Pisces needs to avoid saying, "Don't do that." Gemini is very sensitive and the negative approach will turn him off. In the relationship, apart from sex, Pisces has a calming effect on nervous Gemini. When Pisces is feeling sorry for himself, Gemini is terrific at boosting his spirits.

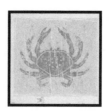

Cancer ~ Cancer
Two Crabs ~ too close for comfort

Cancers are highly emotional people so when the lights are out the sex is terrific, but the relationship is far from paradise. Two of the same Signs together represent a doubling up of all that Sign's inherent qualities, the bad along with the good.

On the positive side, both are highly sexual and enjoy the same amount, duration, and types of sexual behaviors. They have similar timing and strive to satisfy each other. Beyond the bedroom, they share common interests, caring most about family, love, home, and food. They love to shop for antiques, are great bargain hunters, and are generally frugal and quite good with money. Money is important to Cancers and the Crab is usually quite successful. Being an intuitive Water Sign and having a warm personality sets them up to be well liked on the job and to maintain close relationships with their bosses or co-workers.

So the sex can be great and money shouldn't be an issue, but still this is not likely to be a happy couple. Problems surface over matters of control and dominance. Cancer is a controlling Sign and will resent a partner trying to run the show. Cancer also needs to feel loved, and the power struggle with another Cancer is likely to undermine loving feelings. In addition, Cancer has a suspicious streak, which only plays into the tendency to dominate. As both have the same instincts, the result is lack of trust and, at the very least, a difficult relationship to maintain.

SUMMARY

They look into each other's eyes. It's like looking into a mirror or directly into the soul, a feeling that they knew each other in a previous lifetime. The relationship becomes sexual quickly and the sex is hot. With all that promise, sustaining the relationship proves difficult. The struggles between them lead to mistrust, to one trying to control the other, to one watching the other looking for signs of betrayal. And in time there will be betrayal. This relationship is easier if one Cancer is born close to June 23 and the other is born late in the sign, close to July 22.

Cancer ~ Leo
The Crab and the Lion ~ pleasant potential

This combination has plenty of potential though it also has pitfalls. On the positive side, the sex is great. Leo strives to please with gifted hands and mouth. The vitality of Fire Sign Leo excites Cancer. Cancer relies on sensitivity and intuition to know what a lover wants and needs. In addition the loving Water Sign nature of Cancer provides a balance for the Lion's occasionally hyper energy.

Problems crop up when one Sign tries to dominate the other. Leo gives off an aura of competence and willingness to handle considerable responsibility. People always ask Leo to run the show. Since Cancer has a decidedly domineering streak, the Crab won't allow Leo to play King of the Jungle, at least not all the time. Cancer is strong and capable and neither wants nor needs to be ruled. A steady, loving partner is more to the Crab's liking. Also, Leo can be arrogant, which upsets Cancer, and Cancer can be moody, which Leo finds annoying.

Cancer wants attention, in the relationship and out among friends and family, but seldom has the personal magnetism Leo is known for. Just think of their symbols, the noble Lion versus the side-stepping Crab. Cancer is very nice, charming in a quiet way but Leo shines in pubic. Cancer may resent the attention heaped on Leo. The Lion needs to compensate by showering affection on the Crab at home and being mindful of the amount of oxygen he takes up when out in a group.

SUMMARY

Leo is arguably the most powerful sign in the zodiac. Coupled with natural charm and charisma, he is in many ways like the lion symbol of his Sign: the King. Cancer is the Sign of home and food. There is no life without love and food. It's a toss-up as to who is more powerful between these two. But this can be a balance rather than a battlefield as long as there is a clear division of power. And in the bedroom this will be bliss not bloodshed, especially if these two take turns being the top.

Cancer ~ Virgo
The Crab and the Virgin ~ don't worry, be happy

A fine combination. Water Sign Cancer operates from the intuitive, emotional center while Earth Sign Virgo is more pragmatic and logical. Virgo is attentive to detail, a perfectionist, and since Cancer is something of a worrier, this behavior is actually comforting. Both are very social but Cancer has a remarkable capacity to draw people close, in a brief conversation learning all about the other's childhood, current lover, and career. Virgo can spend weeks conversing with people without finding out half this stuff.

Virgo can be fussy and hypercritical and tends to go on and on about a situation. Cancer enjoys listening. When Virgo is hard on himself Cancer is nurturing and accepting. Cancers can be moody and overemotional. Virgo takes this in stride. When they have disagreements, they avoid confrontation. Though not overly significant, there are a few areas of conflict. Virgo has a sarcastic streak and Cancer is easily wounded. Cancer can be too dependent or clingy. Virgo is a strong partner but doesn't want to shoulder all responsibilities.

Both enjoy having sex at least three to four times weekly and like sex to be fairly lengthy. Variety isn't necessary but an experimental range of activities suit both well. They enjoy erotica, some pornography, and using sex toys such as vibrators and dildoes, store bought, hand-carved, or from the produce department at the supermarket. Virgo is all about sensual touch. Cancer represents emotional expressiveness. Their mix of personality traits and behaviors make for great sex and a solid loving relationship.

SUMMARY

As friends or lovers, they communicate and attend to each other's needs intuitively. Cancer is nurturing and emotionally supportive when Virgo is worried and stressed. In return, Virgo provides a feeling of down-to-earth stability. In bed, Cancer's passion and Virgo's willingness to explore make for natural compatibility and gratifying sex. One area of possible concern, Cancer, who is sometimes dependent, may lean on Virgo too heavily. Without being overly critical Virgo must make it clear that he knows Cancer is both strong and capable. In other words, instead of assuming responsibility, Virgo just needs to reassure the Crab.

Cancer ~ Libra
The Crab and the Scales ~ out of balance

One might think that Cancer, Sign of home and family, would be comfortably matched with Libra, Sign of marriage and partnership. But Air Sign Libra, wanting to avoid conflict, sometimes striving for peace at any price, comes across to sensitive Cancer as emotionally detached. Conversely, Libra finds Water Sign Cancer, overly emotional and moody. Yet, when they first meet, Cancer notices Libra's easy elegance, and Libra is drawn to Cancer's warmth and accessibility.

Libra gets turned on by praise, and Cancer is expressive, "I love your body, I love to touch your skin." Cancer wants action, to be kissed and caressed and Libra is an attentive lover. So far so good, but Libra cannot be pushed and takes a long time making decisions. Cancer can be domineering and is given to worry, a quality often triggered by Libra's seeming indecisiveness.

In the bedroom, Libra enjoys a sensual environment with satin sheets, a hint of incense and a well-placed mirror. Cancer, much earthier in nature, less concerned with the setting, enjoys having sex in the woods, near water, and when at home, all that really matters is a modicum of cleanliness. Sex for Libra begins with verbal stimulation, viewing erotica, or phone sex. As to preferences, neither Sign is into sadomasochism but otherwise, almost anything goes with Cancer, including anal penetration. Libra often dislikes anal sex.

Overall, between their personality and sexual differences, it's unlikely for the Scales to find balance or the Crab a happy home in this twosome.

SUMMARY

To start, Cancer will appreciate every part of Libra's body. Libra will reciprocate wanting frequent, hot, heavy sex. But as time passes, Libra, a strong masculine sign, without being overtly aggressive, takes over and runs the show. Cancer is not about to yield and discord ensues. Although Cancer is himself flirtatious, Libra's social charm can be disconcerting to him, even provoking jealousy, which inevitably leads to a show of emotion and hurt. Libra is surprised at Cancer's response since Libra, who isn't given to jealousy, is merely being friendly. Cancer winds up nagging or clinging and Libra wants his freedom.

Cancer ~ **Scorpio**
The Crab and the Scorpion ~ love bites

Two intuitive Water Signs make one great pair. They talk easily about everything, operate out of their emotions, and are sensitive, caring partners. When Cancer is distressed, maybe Scorpio doesn't prod as much as Cancer would like, but Cancer knows that Scorpio can be depended upon.

Cancer is a perplexing Sign, remarkably strong in terms of its nurturing, loving qualities, but also prone to worry. Scorpio's strength is comforting. Scorpio may feel deeply distressed about a problem but doesn't worry. Instead Scorpio focuses on finding solutions. Scorpio has quiet periods and believes that he can work problems out alone. In fact, Scorpio resolves matters far better by bouncing them off someone else. Cancer knows this and patiently strives to draw Scorpio out. Scorpio relishes Cancer's doting nature. Scorpio gets a cold. Cancer makes chicken soup.

Their lovemaking is passionate and so charged with feeling that they experience a sense of oneness. It becomes truly spiritual. Certain sex toys are appealing to secretive Scorpio, namely blindfolds, and Cancer likes to experiment with food. Differences in pace will need accommodating, as Cancer wants sex to last longer than Scorpio. There are also Scorpios for whom rough sex and crude talk are part of the sexual experience, whereas for Cancer that may be a turn-off.

The only relationship problem is that Cancer has a domineering personality and nobody is going to be in charge of Scorpio . . . not for long. Otherwise, this couple has the compatibility to be tremendously successful long term.

SUMMARY

They have a good time together from the beginning, whether out with friends, home alone, or on vacation. While Cancer may be a lot more talkative, Scorpio is a pretty good listener. Scorpio is not put off by Cancer's moodiness. He will shrug his shoulders and go for a walk. He is good at comforting Cancer when Cancer is worried and enjoys the fact that Cancer loves the role of doting, nurturing partner. In the bedroom, Cancer wants more foreplay and Scorpio wants more variety, otherwise their lovemaking is as easy and comfortable as all other aspects of their relationship.

Cancer ~ Sagittarius
The Crab and the Archer ~ tough-going but possible

Cancer's motto is "Home Sweet Home." Sagittarius says, "Don't fence me in." Cancer's symbol, the Crab, is a creature that moves sideways, a creature that is cautious and stays inside its own home. Sagittarius is the Archer, whose arrow flies straight to its mark. In other words, Cancer has a sensitive, self-protective nature while Sagittarius is at times reckless and always direct, to the point of bluntness. Without intending to hurt, Sagittarius's words leave their mark and Cancer, with a remarkable memory, will bear the scars forever.

The beginning is fun. Cancer is excited by the broad and expansive ideas of Sagittarius. Sagittarius is turned on by the warmth and attentiveness of Cancer. They have a great time together in public. Cancer is a bit reticent. Sagittarius is self-assured. Both are passionate and intense lovers, highly oral, and each will strive to impress the other.

They can be great friends and in business these two could balance each other very well. Cancer would hold down the home base, and Sagittarius would be out in the field dealing with the public. The personal relationship is harder to sustain.

Sagittarius has an aura of cool detachment or aloofness, which can trigger insecurity and resentment in Cancer. Cancer will try in all ways possible to entice the Archer into staying within home territory. Neither would be long satisfied. Even thought the sex can be terrific, they are opposites in goals and temperaments, and these fundamental differences make sustaining this relationship long-term very tough.

SUMMARY

Want to travel? Sagittarius is the perfect man. Try to coop him up and he's history. Cancer dotes. Sagittarius withdraws. The Archer loves a good debate. Cancer is hurt by the vehemence of the argument. The beginning is as exciting as it gets. The ending may be equally explosive. Sagittarius doesn't mean to hurt Cancer, but Cancer won't let go. Sag says, "You're too good for me." Cancer should believe him and move on. These two are best advised to enjoy the friendship, the company, and the travels. Enjoy the sex, it will be exhilarating. In the morning, go separate ways.

Cancer ~ Capricorn
The Crab and the Goat ~ opposites attract and repel

As a business combination, the balance of Cancer intuition and Capricorn practicality is fine. A long-term romantic relationship is more difficult. Cancerian mottoes include, "Home is where the heart is. A man's home is his castle," and "The way to a man's heart is through his stomach." Capricorn thinks, "Don't hang your dirty linens in public. Keep your cards close to your chest," and wonders, "What will the neighbors think?"

If this couple has enough money to paint either the interior or the exterior of their house but not both, Cancer would paint the inside and Capricorn the outside. For Capricorn the well-kept house projects an image of success. For Cancer, an inviting atmosphere, the smells of cinnamon and coffee, and the welcome mat at the front door are far more important.

Cancer is sensitive, intuitive, and perhaps the most emotional of all the Signs. Capricorn is pragmatic, matter-of-fact, takes a logical approach, and tends to be reserved. Both can be controlling and neither takes that well. Cancer would respond with moodiness. Capricorn would be manipulative.

Sex starts out great and, if both work at keeping the physical relationship healthy, that will go far to help this twosome stay together. Their sex life begins with lots of intensity, both like it to last for thirty minutes to an hour and they like the same range of behaviors. Over time, however, even in their sex life, Cancer finds Capricorn to be distant and Capricorn thinks Cancer is too emotional.

SUMMARY

This isn't an easy combo but it can work. The opposite qualities of these Signs may create successful balances for each other. Capricorn tends to be guarded, cautious in relationships. Cancer wades right in. As a result, Cancer warms up Capricorn, opening up his affectionate side. Capricorn helps Cancer to develop a thicker skin and be less emotionally reactive. Capricorn is a natural leader in the business world while Cancer rules the roost. As long as Capricorn mixes affection with his sexual behaviors, this part of their relationship will be highly successful. It's living together that's apt to be trying.

Cancer ~ Aquarius
The Crab and the Water Bearer ~
if not passion, contentment

Most often when a Water Sign like Cancer connects with an Air Sign like Aquarius, you get steam . . . a whole lot of instant reaction, dissipated rapidly into nothingness. Surprise! This pair has the potential to be a good combination, though it won't be easy.

For Aquarius, Cancer provides warmth, open affection, and commitment, qualities that comfort Aquarius who is well mannered, diplomatic, friendly, and yet emotionally detached. For Cancer, it's the brilliance of the Aquarian mind, the social aspect with people around all the time, and the amount of variety Aquarius always has in life that are so appealing.

Cancer is a bit of a homebody and Aquarius wants to be out and about. Finding ways to satisfy each other requires compromise, hitting the clubs on Saturday and sharing a pizza and watching a video on Sunday.

Sex is an area of potential difficulty. Cancer may be willing to experiment with some sex toys and a few costumes, some food in the sex play, but not much more than that. Overall, Cancer's approach to sex is about deep feelings of intimacy and passion. Aquarius, seeking sensation, wants to probe deeper into fetishes, which is not necessarily a comfortable foray for Cancer. Aquarius is more about observing, experimenting, and exploring new territory. "Lets try that toy and see how it feels." Cancer may be dissatisfied and Aquarius does not comprehend what's missing.

If these two strive to overcome the problems in the bedroom, they can sustain a contented and respectful, albeit not overly passionate, relationship.

SUMMARY

Cancer is fascinated by Aquarius's diplomatic ability to mix with senators and street people and remain even-tempered under stress. Cancer is emotional and moody but Aquarius recognizes Cancer's loving devotion. Not an easy relationship, although the attraction suggests it's worth the struggle. For sexual satisfaction beyond initial lust, Aquarius must be more affectionate and Cancer more open to experimentation. Taking turns accepting responsibility for setting the stage and creating the scene for sex will pay off. Aquarius might dim the lights and provide incense. Cancer would perform a little telephone sex earlier in the day or supply a new toy.

Cancer ~ Pisces
The Crab and the Fish ~ true love lasting forever

Frequently when two Water Signs get together, all you get is drenched. Where's the substance of Earth, the vitality of Fire, or the stimulus of Air? With these two, no such problem exists. Cancer and Pisces make for a playground romance. The affection and the shared emotions represent the typical, "falling in love, living in the little house in the woods happily ever after" fairytale relationship.

Cancer wants the all-American dream lifestyle, a house to call his own, a patch of ground to grow some vegetables or flowers, a dog to take for a walk, and the stereotypical white picket fence. Pisces shares that dream and extends it out from their private half acre into the community. They make a loving couple, have a very gratifying sex life and most of the time are very in sync with each other.

Okay, there can be problems. Sometimes Cancer gets crabby and moody. Pisces has an occasional bout of self-pity. If there should be an argument, Pisces will seem to yield and Cancer believes they've come to an agreement. All too often, however, Pisces has just stopped arguing and may go right on doing whatever he wants. Simply put, Pisces can't be pushed, cajoled perhaps, but know this, fighting with Pisces is like punching a rubber wall . . . walk away and the wall just resumes its previous condition.

These two are so well suited, however, that they work through tough and touchy periods. This is truly the couple that can look forward to celebrating decades together.

SUMMARY

Natural friends, business partners, and lovers, these two have a lustful time in bed and a lasting relationship. When Cancer frets and worries, Pisces listens sympathetically. When Pisces feels offended by the cruelties of the world, Cancer soothes with his nurturing ways, loving words, or a massage. Pisces enjoys romance and fantasies of exotic places. It may never have been his thing, but Cancer will get into role-playing. At the worst, Cancer's cloying behavior may occasionally annoy Pisces, and Pisces's self-pitying may upset Cancer. But neither problem occurs often and both get past small grievances without rancor or holding grudges.

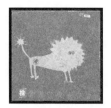

Leo ~ Leo
Two Lions together ~ fire, fire burning bright

Fire Sign Leo is open, direct, personable, and easy to get along with, if one remembers that Leo is always right. Really, Leo is right most of the time. But when Leo is wrong, the Lion still prefers the other person to apologize. Put two Leos together and there will be occasions when both are right but have different opinions. In the big picture this is a tough relationship to sustain, but the benefits are worth the effort.

Leo is a performer, needs an audience and, when given attention and praise, reciprocates with generosity. In public, each enjoys holding court, which might lead to competition, but more often than not, generosity of spirit prevails. This Sign is also extravagant but fortunate, so money need not be a problem.

Leo is such a competent Sign that others frequently ask them to assume responsibilities at work and in the community. Leo has a hard time saying "no" and with so many activities outside the home, may have less than adequate energy to attend to a partner, which won't suit Leo #2 at all.

Their sex life is great, experimental in range, including dominance and submission, having sex in public places, voyeurism. They also enjoy ménage à trois, and incorporating food. Leo likes sex often and approach the act with intensity. It's a mark of pride to please his partner. Leos share similar interests and are active people who enjoy being out with friends, traveling, attending concerts and movies. Overall, their life together can be passionate, rewarding, and fun.

SUMMARY

Can you imagine two kings of the jungle, two strong personalities, living under the same roof? Intense and passionate, the future can be successful with a degree of effort and attention. Without doubt, this relationship will go through periods of trouble. Each needs so much in the way of attention, affection, and admiration. To make this combo work long-term, one Leo has to assume greater responsibility for managing the money, as both are given to extravagance and both Leos must be able to shrug off the other's exaggerated sense of self-importance. It helps that they share a delightful sense of humor.

Leo ~ Virgo
The Lion and the Virgin ~ an odd couple

Leo is sort of sloppy where Virgo can be too neat. Long term they aggravate each other. Virgo is always picking on Leo for things that Leo finds inconsequential. Leo says, "So what?" Put these two between the sheets, however, and it's quite fine. Leo, the actor, enjoys Virgo, the director, saying "a little to the left, a little to the right."

Their differences are many. Leo has an optimistic attitude in life, "I'm an open book, you can know everything about me because I'm wonderful." The Lion is dynamic, extravagant, and a risk-taker. Virgo is cautious, not volunteering much personal information until feeling quite secure in a relationship. Virgo is a discriminating, hard-working, and dependable friend.

Virgo is slightly flirtatious, Leo is over the top. Both Signs are highly sexual with different preferences. Risk taking Leo enjoys voyeurism and sex in public places. Virgo would prefer to do it rather than watch it, and he wants to have sex in the quiet safety of his own home.

Leo needs to be adored. A sexual turn-on for Leo is being praised during foreplay and the act itself. Virgo is short on compliments. Leos want to be trusted, not questioned, by their partner. Virgo questions everything. Virgos want appreciation for the hard work and effort that they put into the relationship. Leo doesn't see why it should be so much work. Over the years the contrast between these two personalities makes this combo difficult to sustain in any meaningful and fulfilling way.

SUMMARY

Leo sees himself as the natural leader and expects everyone in his sphere to agree. This doesn't fly with Virgo. At work Virgo may be content to be second in command, but in a relationship he wants equality. Money is another area of potential conflict. Leo is extravagant and one of anything is never enough. If he has two bucks he buys two television sets. If he has $2,000 he buys two pickup trucks. Virgo wants to be sure that all the bills can be paid. Initially the sex will be hot and heavy, no-holds-barred, but sustaining this relationship is very difficult.

Leo ~ Libra
The Lion and the Scales ~ cozy balance

Fire Signs like Leo and Air Signs like Libra are generally a harmonious match. Libra loves Leo's exuberance. Leo is turned on by Libra's style and gentle disposition. Libra wants a steadfast partner who is also independent. Cuddling is great but space is necessary. Libra wants to be free to roam around, be admired, and flirt. Leo is okay with this as long as it is obviously just playful; the Lion has a jealous streak. But Libra knows this and is attentive to the Lion as well.

Leo wants a loyal, devoted audience and has that in Libra who is delighted by Leo's sense of humor. They take pleasure in having a well-tended house and yard, though they prefer to have someone else do the tending. They are both spontaneous, "Let's pack our bags and take off for the weekend." Neither is overly critical or demanding.

Sex is comfortable, whether it lasts an hour or five minutes, sometimes passionate, always satisfying. Both like sex ranging into the experimental, some role-playing, a bit of dominance and submission, and a little food in the mix. The setting is more important to Libra but Leo is willing to accommodate.

Money may be a problem. Leo is extravagant and Libra is the Sign of luxury. They want to live well. So Leo's exuberance in buying the latest technological gizmo or plasma TV best be matched by his income, and Libra's acquisitive streak must also be balanced with matching funds or there will be serious disagreements.

SUMMARY

Conversation is easy and satisfying. They enjoy doing similar things, traveling, gambling, just strolling by the lake. Leo is the dominant male in the relationship, not always in the bedroom. With anal sex, for example, Libra may be the top. Their sexual behaviors are similar and sex is generally satisfying. It does take a little more effort to put Libra in the mood. Leo's always ready. If sex isn't perfect, Leo will stay in the relationship, whereas Libra will be out charming some other guy in short order. A little compromise and just the right dildo might save this relationship.

Leo ~ Scorpio
The Lion and the Scorpion ~ an uphill battle

This pairing is difficult, both Signs are strong-headed and obstinate, but the relationship has a chance. Scorpio and Leo are fixed Signs and they have profound respect for each other. Scorpio brings devotion to the relationship. Leo brings enthusiasm. Leo admires Scorpio's resourcefulness, while Scorpio finds Leo's natural leadership ability and charm highly appealing. Sexually, they're both very passionate and open to a fair range of sexual exploration, though Scorpio may be more open than Leo. Scorpio strives to satisfy Leo by staying attuned to him. Leo gets very carried away. Scorpio enjoys the excursion and is content to let Leo lead, at least in the bedroom.

But their differences are vast. Leo is outgoing, direct, flamboyant, self-assured, and can be arrogant. Scorpio is guarded and reserved and cannot begin to match Leo's bottomless self-confidence. In fact, Scorpio envies it and strives to learn from it. Leo wants Scorpio to take more chances. Scorpio wants Leo to calm down some. A strong sense of humor is an invaluable asset.

In the relationship the biggest problem, from Leo's point of view, is Scorpio's stubbornness. As Scorpio sees it, Leo is temperamental and demanding. Leo likes to be right. In fact, Leo is convinced that he is always right. Scorpio may adore Leo and be willing to concede most of the time, but not always. If, over time, Scorpio becomes more confrontational, less willing to concede, Leo is liable to turn off and the sex life could die out.

SUMMARY

A better friendship or business partnership than love affair, these two respect each other but are inherently so different. Leo has a natural exuberance for life, a winning personality that draws people to him. Scorpio has an aura of intrigue or mystery, compelling but also disconcerting. Scorpio may view Leo as having a self-inflated image, because Scorpio tends to put himself down, which Leo never does. The sexual energy between these two is intense initially, but here too the differences outweigh the similarities. The only way for this relationship to last through time is if they live by the credo "vive la difference."

Leo ~ Sagittarius
The Lion and the Archer ~ play time

This combination is playful and great sexually. Two Fire Signs together can be explosive, as this element is known for wanting to dominate all relationships, but Leo and Sagittarius are successful because Sagittarius is the least aggressive of the Fire Signs, and is, in fact, pretty mellow.

In all aspects of life, sex included, Leo is energetic, vital, and enthusiastic. Even the most sophisticated, mature, seemingly controlled Leo has a playful quality. Sagittarius is dazzled, charmed, and smitten. Sagittarius is the philosopher of the zodiac, with a remarkable ability to take a long view of life, while Leo is acquisitive, the quintessential consumer, all involved in the moment. Each finds the other's outlook intriguing. In the bedroom, Sagittarius wants to impress Leo with force and duration in lovemaking. Leo responds with fervor and intensity. Whether mainstream or more experimental in range of sexuality, each will find a willing partner in the other.

There are a couple of problems. Sagittarius speaks his mind without thinking through the effect of those words. Leo is easily wounded. Also, Sagittarius resents Leo's attitude of always being right. A problem area for Leo: Sagittarius is the gambler of the zodiac and not above cutting corners to achieve his ends. Leo may tell an occasional lie, to the extent that anybody will, but Leo is by nature honest and adamant about principles.

In spite of these problems, the Lion and the Archer are fundamentally well suited and likely to share a happy long-lasting relationship.

SUMMARY

For Sagittarius "Don't fence me in" is fundamental. Sagittarius won't put up with possessiveness. He is both restless and physical, and may enjoy hiking, tennis, or horseback riding. Leo may be the dominant male but he isn't truly controlling. He enjoys sharing Sagittarius's activities. As long as Leo remains aware of his tendency to behave like "the man in charge," the Archer will be content. Both men are likely to have had extensive sexual experiences. If Leo asks, Sagittarius will most likely report in detail. Leo will be bothered by this knowledge long after. This is clearly a case for "don't ask, don't tell."

Leo ~ Capricorn
The Lion and the Goat ~ unnatural pairing

Capricorn is reserved, where Leo is expressive, frugal where Leo is extravagant, and pragmatic where Leo is both optimistic and trusting. Capricorn represents the work ethic, Leo trusts luck. They may respect each other and have a loving friendship, but their fundamental differences are vast and over the long haul this remains a tough combination.

Imagine going to a large party. Somewhere in the middle of the room one person stands surrounded by a group. That's Leo, the center of attention, holding forth with charming stories, the actor's delivery, and a captivating personality. In another part of the room is a striking figure, stately, composed, calm, quiet, and also compelling. Capricorn notices Leo and finds Leo's energy sexually exciting. After Leo tires of entertaining the crowd, he notices Capricorn and is equally drawn.

As soon as Leo recognizes that the attraction is mutual, Leo is ready for the main event. No way, not with Capricorn. The Goat trusts his instincts and may get sexual soon but very seldom on a first encounter, and trying to rush him will have the opposite effect. If Leo hangs out for a while and impresses Capricorn sufficiently, they'll find some place more private.

Initially the sex can be great. Over time, Capricorn wants to take it slow, Leo moves fast, undermining the sexual expression. They may like the same behaviors, but from foreplay to orgasm, their pace and timing are at odds. Sadly, the lack of sparks will ultimately kill the relationship.

SUMMARY

Here we have Leo, fundamentally flirtatious, and Capricorn, who is relatively quiet and subtle. Both can be jealous. If Leo isn't the center of attention his feelings of jealousy get triggered. If Capricorn thinks that he's being made a fool, his pride will be wounded. In fact, the worst thing one can do to Leo is ignore him, and the worst thing one can do to Capricorn is wound his pride. The way that they communicate is also at odds. Leo is talkative. Capricorn keeps things to himself. Even in the bedroom, once the initial lust fades there is little satisfaction.

Leo ~ Aquarius
The Lion and the Water Bearer ~ opposites attract and repel

Aquarius's dignity and wonderful conversation skills charm Leo. The Water Bearer, preferring to observe, stays somewhat on the sidelines, enjoying flirting and talking quietly. Aquarius is drawn to the open vibrancy of Leo for whom all the world's a stage, with the Lion very much in its center.

The relationship they form is cordial and in business or friendship can be satisfying. On the personal level, they do not bring out the best in each other. Aquarius feels unappreciated as Leo is so focused on his own activities. Leo finds Aquarius emotionally detached. Sex for Aquarius starts with verbal seduction made early in the day. Anticipation is heightened by sexy phone chats later. All this talk about sex gets tedious for Leo who just wants to do something. By the time Aquarius is through talking about sex, Leo is too tired.

Leo is concerned about being forthright. Aquarius tempers his words to the situation. Think of Aquarius as the ambassador, sent to the hot spots of the world to mediate. It's a good thing that he can keep cool and chooses his words with care. But Leo comes to distrust this seemingly cagey quality.

Leo is the Sign of summer, ruled by the Sun, all hot and fiery. Aquarius is a Winter Sign, cool, crisp, and emotionally reserved. These two are as different as fire and ice and their personalities, especially in intimate relationships, make this a very uneasy coupling. As Sun Signs pairs go, these two make among the most difficult of combinations.

SUMMARY

The attraction is instant and powerful, the first few encounters lustful. Long-term the potential is dim. Leo wants peace and quiet at home, a partner who is giving and loving. Aquarius is restless and ever looking for new activities. Aquarius is too cool, too cerebral to satisfy Leo's passionate nature. Conversely, the Water Bearer finds Leo's intensity exhausting. Sexually, a long verbal buildup gets Aquarius going. For Leo, everything is spontaneous. Aquarius comes to find Leo's approach routine and Leo finds Aquarius's need for variety too much like work. The relationship is unlikely to last, but these two Signs do make great friends.

Leo ~ Pisces
The Lion and the Fish ~ incompatible species

Initially, this is a fun thing. Pisces is such a romantic and so good at giving praise, Leo is delighted. The sex is passionate and Pisces, with a strong constitution, keeps things going a lot longer than is the usual case with Leo. Pisces with great imagination brings new elements to lovemaking, incense, candles, and different settings. Both Signs are quite experimental in sexual range, enjoying sex in public places, using costumes, leather or latex, and get turned on by sexy underwear. Leo also finds tattoos and shaved genitals exciting. Pisces likes to use hot wax and ice cubes in sex play and may well have a foot fetish. If sex is the beginning and the end between these two, all's well. As a relationship, troubles lie ahead.

Leo is a powerful Sign, willing to confront problems head on. Pisces is a strong Sign, it is the Sign of medicine and healing, but the Fish is not confrontational. Pisces depends upon negotiating skill, quiet maneuvering, doing what is needed as a matter of expediency to get what he wants. Leo sees this as a lack of scruples and gets turned off.

Pisces has a need for retreat, for time to meditate. Leo may feel shut out. The Fish also has short periods of self-pity with which Leo has no patience. The Lion is all about action, often precipitously. Pisces is all about intuition and makes decisions based on belief and instinct. Neither is overly pragmatic. Life's mundane details undermine their stability as a couple.

SUMMARY

Sex, whether in the bedroom with creature comforts or in some public place, is passionate and fulfilling, but beyond that for two creatures as different as the Lion and the Fish, there is little common ground. Leo is very social, enjoys active dates, such as miniature golf, bowling, camping, and being out with many friends. Pisces prefers a quieter lifestyle, entertaining at home, going for leisurely strolls rather than hiking a mountain trail. Leo is more impulsive, acting on inspiration, while Pisces is more introspective and thoughtful in decision-making. There is little satisfaction for one with the other over time.

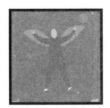

Virgo ~ Virgo
Two Virgins together ~ let's try that again

Put two Virgos together and you've got a kind of tape recorder specialist on sexual relations. They get it all down and replay it over and over, testing and analyzing who's outperforming whom, and in their minds, they're having fun. After all, Virgo is a perfectionist wanting to do everything right. So when Virgo gives directions—"do more of this, no, no, more to the right, yes, that feels wonderful"—all goes fairly well in the bedroom. But there can be a problem because, between these two, there is no spark, no unexpected energy.

Sexually, this is a Sign that comes in two extremes. The more mainstream Virgo enjoys oral and anal sex, ménage à trois, and a variety of sex toys, including dildoes, cock rings, vibrators, and butt plugs. The more open Virgo is into bondage, dominance, and submission and occasionally sadomasochism.

Doubling up the good qualities of Virgo, practicality, directness, willingness to work hard and be supportive is fine. Doubling up on the negative qualities, nitpicking, needing to examine and reexamine all things, becomes tedious. And while Virgo is a highly critical Sign, Virgo doesn't take criticism well. The good news is that these problems are surmountable. Virgo/Virgo can make for a very successful couple. Each needs to guard against being overly fault-finding. Both need to let some matters go without extensive rehashing.

Two Virgos can have a very satisfying relationship, being supportive of each other and great friends. However, if their sex drives are very mismatched, the relationship is likely to fail.

SUMMARY

This couple is most successful if one Virgo is seven years or so older than the other. Virgo tends to think he knows exactly how things should be done. He is a hard-working perfectionist and expects a fair reward for his effort. With age he learns life doesn't necessarily work this way. Therefore the older Virgo will be more understanding and more tolerant when the younger Virgo rails against the slings and arrows of outrageous fortune. Of course, in bed, the younger Virgo may have a trick or two to teach the older one, and there are always new toys to try.

Virgo ~ Libra
The Virgin and the Scales ~ an uneasy imbalance

These two are fine as friends or business partners, but as lovers they're mismatched in bed and out. Though good-hearted, Virgo is given to complaining and nit-picking, which is hurtful to Libra. Libra enjoys chattering about almost anything while Virgo is not long on small talk. On the positive side, both strive to avoid confrontation. It violates Libra's gentle, polite nature and innate struggle for balance, and it's at odds with the Virgin's cool, objective, analytical approach to problem-solving.

Regarding sex, Virgo generally programs everything, including the time and place, and follows a set process from foreplay to climax. Earth Sign Virgo is turned on by touch and spends lots of time during foreplay exploring a partner's body with inquisitive and exciting fingers. Sometimes Virgo likes to get down and dirty with raunchy sex talk and the use of pornography.

Libra, an Air Sign, needs verbal set up to get into the mood. The more sexy talk, tantalizing not crude, the readier he is. Libra dislikes anything harsh, is far less structured, prefers spontaneity, and likes oral play—kissing, licking, sucking—more than extensive touching.

Sex may work out better if these two explore some fetishes and experiment with a variety of sex toys. Libra's interest in sex may be greater in the area of fetishistic role-playing accoutrements than Virgo, but Virgo is curious and usually willing to try new things. Virgo needs to remember that Libra wants romance. A compromise between these two may be difficult but could also be a lot of fun.

SUMMARY

Virgo finds one right way to do it, whatever it is. Libra does it several different ways. Virgo wonders why Libra complicates life that way and becomes critical. Libra takes offense. Libra has a lazy streak. Virgo works at everything . . . including sex. He directs it and prepares for it with props. Libra wants to play, be romanced, and praised, where Virgo is matter-of-fact. Virgo likes to draw sex out. Libra wants to build up to it at dinner or on a long walk and in the bedroom go right to the heart of the matter. Staying together will always require effort.

Virgo ~ Scorpio
The Virgin and the Scorpion ~ the sting becomes a love tap

This is a great combination. There's natural chemistry that draws these two together in a bond that grows over time into mutual respect. Virgo and Scorpio share a quiet, almost subterranean, connection that provides comfort for both. They can talk about anything and rarely upset each other. Virgo is down to earth, straightforward, and direct. With Virgo, what you see is what you get, qualities that Scorpio admires. For Virgo, who has a tendency to worry, Scorpio is steadying and reassuring.

The sex will be comfortable, even quite passionate as Scorpio knows how to energize Virgo, to get Virgo to let go of the structured or predictable and become more spontaneous. Conversely, Virgo knows how to prolong the experience and tease Scorpio to greater heights. Virgo wants sex frequently, it's good for one's health, and Scorpio is glad to oblige. Both Signs enjoy the thrill of sex in public places, exhibitionism, and using a variety of sex toys. They strive to reach orgasm together and climax virtually every time they have sex.

Scorpio appreciates Virgo's work ethic, on the job, at home, and in his social life. Where Virgo may suffer from feelings of self-doubt, Scorpio's profound strength is comforting. Virgo is wonderful about assisting a partner to achieve his goals. Scorpio is good at encouraging Virgo to stretch for new objectives. Virgo is not put off by Scorpio's silences and Scorpio does not object to Virgo's fussiness. In fact, trait for trait, both are accepting and comfortable with the other's little quirks.

SUMMARY

The foundation is friendship and respect. Virgo always comes through for his friends, without waiting to be asked, without expecting a pat on the back. Scorpio admires that quality as well as Virgo's earnest desire to please. Virgo admires Scorpio's intensity and single mindedness of purpose. Virgo wants to open up sexually and responds to Scorpio's passion. Their only problem is that when Virgo gets into a satisfactory sexual routine, he stays with it, unchanging. Scorpio finds any routine boring, especially in the bedroom. Generally speaking the potential is good for sex that is comforting, consistent, and tender, if not exciting.

Virgo ~ Sagittarius
The Virgin and the Archer ~ mixed metaphor

This relationship represents a conflict physically and emotionally. Sagittarius takes a rather breezy approach to love and sex. Virgo is very serious, a perfectionist, even about lovemaking. Both Signs like to spend about one hour having sex, but they spend this time very differently. Sagittarius wants to romanticize sex, to drag it out, make it interesting, discuss it, whereas Virgo wants to focus squarely on the sex. Virgo wants time to run his hands over every inch of the Sagittarius body. The passion of Sagittarius is turned off by this almost analytical exploration.

Virgo is the worker of the zodiac. Sagittarius is the philosopher. Virgo attends to all details, while Sagittarius takes the long view. Work for Virgo is getting things done. Work for Sagittarius may be thinking things through. Virgo is mature at an early age, ready to accept considerable responsibility even while still a teenager. Sagittarius struggles to find balance between freedom and responsibility. In the younger years Sagittarius avoids responsibility fearing it will limit freedom. Later on Sagittarius becomes very responsible but never gives up the quest for fun and pleasure.

Virgo will have to make a terrific effort to remember hearts and flowers, violins, and the gentle scent of vanilla to keep Sagittarius happy in the bedroom. Sagittarius will have to be more focused and help Virgo with the nitty-gritty aspects of life to make this relationship last more than a short while. Fundamentally, Virgo feels threatened and insecure with Sagittarius, and Sagittarius feels stifled by Virgo.

SUMMARY

This is not a comfortable twosome. As personalities, they don't meet each other's needs. Sagittarius doesn't care about things that Virgo considers important. Virgo says, "Let's do it now." Sagittarius asks, "What's the big deal?" Virgo feels brushed aside. Sex is the best part of this relationship. Sagittarius is famous for being well endowed and proud of his equipment. As long as Virgo shows that he's mightily impressed, he'll keep a Sagittarius interested. In bed, the main problem is that Virgo is too stuck in routine and Sagittarius wants more variety. Virgo wants true love. Sagittarius wants every lover.

Virgo ~ Capricorn
The Virgin and the Goat ~ add a little spice

This is not a passionate love affair but rather a stable relationship that can last through time. Virgo and Capricorn have a great deal in common. They enjoy traveling, talking, and working together. They're down to earth, practical, and have respect for order. Virgo is a remarkably loyal partner as is Capricorn. They both expect a lot of themselves and therefore from their partners.

In the bedroom, what starts out great can get dull. Initially they enjoy exploring each other's bodies, and they both have fabulous hands with which they make the whole body an erogenous zone. Still over time, this sex play, lacking in spontaneity, can become predictable and unexciting. Going outside the mainstream will spice up their sex life.

Remember, though Virgo is known as the Virgin Sign, many Virgos are into exploring physical stimulus and sensations far beyond mainstream oral and anal sex. Could it be that their puritanical outer behavior hides a lustful interior that almost embarrasses them? Without doubt, they are quiet about their secret wild bedroom excursions. In Capricorn this Virgo finds a willing partner.

Capricorn likes experimental sex. Still, introducing such things as the subject of bondage, discipline, and sadomasochism must be done with care. This is the couple who may enjoy exploring sexual role-playing and the entire BDSM lifestyle. For one thing, Virgos like to be spanked. They are perfectionists. Perhaps they expect spankings when their performance is less than perfect. Capricorn, the master, the military general, is all too ready to administer the punishment.

SUMMARY

Potential soul mates. Virgo won't seduce Capricorn on the first night. Capricorn wants to develop a friendship and some understanding of a man's mind before exploring his body. An ideal evening for these two would be quiet, away from the club scene, a stroll along the beach or a conversation in front of the fireplace. There are distinct roles here. Capricorn is the leader, though not conspicuously. Virgo enjoys serving. All this works in the bedroom as long as role-playing and sex toys are added to the repertoire. Otherwise, as time passes, the sexual connection, though satisfying, will be unexciting.

Virgo ~ Aquarius
The Virgin and the Water Bearer ~ but how do you feel?

This combination is most successful as a friendship. Both are slow to reveal much about their private lives. Virgo wants to be sure that a developing relationship could become more than a casual acquaintanceship before opening up. Aquarius doesn't reveal personal information.

Major problems for these two stem from the arena of emotion. Virgo may feel things intensely but isn't expressive. Aquarius operates from intellect and inspiration rather than from feelings. Therefore, when there are relationship problems, Virgo chooses to analyze them in depth, while Aquarius wants to discuss things at length, but neither is comfortable getting at the emotional underpinnings. In time what's left is a polite, well-mannered life without much warmth.

Sexually these two are decidedly mismatched. Sexy talk is enough to put Aquarius on the edge of orgasm. Virgo needs a fair amount of foreplay to reach that plateau. In one way sex can work for this couple if Virgo is open to experimenting with behaviors beyond vanilla sex. Aquarius is often willing to try fetishes, role-playing, and the use of toys and equipment in sexual behaviors. Even though the motive is sensation, as opposed to being carried away with passion, the result can be exciting lovemaking for both.

There is such a difference between the raw, earthy sexuality of Virgo and the intellectual sexuality of Aquarius. Virgo may seem so cut and dry in his demeanor, but he has a passionate heart. Aquarius seems so upbeat and outgoing, but at the core he remains detached. They don't bring out the best in each other.

SUMMARY

From the beginning they communicate with each other easily and a solid friendship develops. They share intellectual interests and as partners manage to handle responsibilities fairly. For these reasons they can live together comfortably. Unfortunately, they are not well suited in the bedroom. While both enjoy frequent sex, their turn-ons and choice of behaviors are at odds. In addition, Aquarius wants to get to the heart of the matter very quickly. Virgo wants time for his hands to explore every inch of the delightful Aquarius physique. Long term, this sexual disparity is likely to be destructive to the relationship.

Virgo ~ Pisces
The Virgin and the Fish ~ worth getting your feet wet

Virgo and Pisces, opposite Signs, both attract and repel. Virgo provides stability and down-to-earth, day-by-day practicality. Pisces provides emotional warmth and sexual intensity. Pisces is highly spiritual. Virgo is matter-of-fact. This attraction is hard to sustain because the emotional world Pisces inhabits, while fascinating to Virgo, is also overwhelming, so much so that Virgo may leave. And yet, the sex could be so good that it would be well worth the effort to sustain the relationship and get through difficult times.

When Virgo feels stressed and has the tendency to go on and on, when Pisces feels unfairly attacked and retreats into self-pity, it is important to remember that Virgo is a steadfast supportive friend and Pisces a loving partner.

Virgo is not usually an aggressive sign, comfortable having someone else in the director's position. However, with Pisces, which is such a flexible Sign, Virgo may become domineering. When there's a disagreement, Virgo enjoys a good debate, but Pisces retreats from them. Then Virgo believes a resolution has been achieved, when in fact, Pisces has merely stopped arguing without necessarily conceding.

Those Virgos who are more experimental or open in their lovemaking prove to be easier mates for passionate Pisces. Their sex life will be enhanced by adding costumes, leather and latex, perhaps bondage, or trying a ménage à trois. In fact, in this twosome, Virgo will have free rein to explore all the kinkiness that he desires, as Pisces likes to act out sex fantasies. And Pisces will certainly appreciate a foot massage.

SUMMARY

The sex will be wonderful in lengthy lovemaking sessions or brief ones. Virgo enjoys exploring his partner's body with his hands, while Pisces reciprocates with his mouth. Outside the bedroom, Pisces is by nature flirtatious but means nothing by it. Virgo has a tendency to feel jealous. He must learn to overlook this fundamental quality in Pisces for the sake of the relationship. Other problems arise from Virgo trying to run the show. While Pisces isn't aggressive, neither is he anyone's pushover. If he finds Virgo overly dominant, he'll simply do what he wants, which may undermine trust between them.

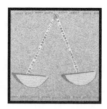

Libra ~ Libra
The Scales with the Scales ~ yes, no, well, maybe

Venus, planet of love and beauty, harmony, and elegance rules Libra. Libra hates people who are demanding, loud, and crude in public. Two such kind, truly nice individuals should make a wonderful twosome. Not necessarily.

Libra strives to avoid confrontations, backing away from touchy issues, even denying a problem exists. Unfortunately denial doesn't make things better. Time passes, frustrations build, and the day comes when out pours a lengthy list of remembered grievances, creating great distress as the list includes many items that were supposedly of no concern. For this relationship to succeed, both must face problems when they arise.

Libra is reputedly indecisive. That's not accurate. Rather, Libra sees many possibilities and needs to weigh and measure them before making a choice, because having chosen, Libra will stick to that position. It does, therefore, take Libra a long time to make a decision. Two Libras have a doubly difficult time settling on a course of action whether the decision is minor, "Your place or mine?" or major, "Should we buy a house, which one, should we start a business?" Over time this behavior proves tedious and creates a state of confusion, of emotional instability, and the sex, therefore, doesn't produce much satisfaction.

In fact, in the bedroom, after the initial heat of an affair passes, it isn't easy to keep the spark going. Perhaps the best way for this couple to maintain excitement in their sex life is to have other partners on the side, or enter a ménage à trois arrangement.

SUMMARY

Libra loves beauty. He spots an elegant man across a crowded room and is drawn to his side. Of course, this handsome man is a Libra. With charm, not aggression, with a delightful sense of humor, Libra attracts attention. The love affair starts quickly. Sexually almost anything goes, except crudeness. Try to force anything on a Libra and one discovers a pronounced stubborn streak. These two can be great friends, but in an intimate relationship as they have almost too much in common, including the same faults, feelings fade. The lazy streak and tendency to self-indulgence are likely to undermine this relationship.

Libra ~ Scorpio
The Scales and the Scorpion ~ mixed metaphor

Initially ardent, it is soon obvious that their styles are distinctly different, leading ultimately to lukewarm sex and an unsatisfying relationship. Signs that come side by side, as Libra and Scorpio do, seldom complement each other.

Libra, genuinely nice, gentle, and good-natured, seeks to avoid strife, is refined and also self-indulgent. Scorpio, intense, driven, and relentless, will not back away from a confrontation, and they seldom ever describe themselves as "nice." They might think of themselves as good, committed, and caring, but nice isn't an adjective that fits. Scorpios have fierce tempers. They want intensity, emotion and passion in their lives. Libra is even-tempered and strives for a life of contentment. Libra wants to go out with friends to movies, sports events, flower shows. Scorpio is often content to stay at home, focused on some project or other.

When it comes to sex, most Librans are true to their Sign. They want sex to be something lofty, elegant, not too sweaty or messy. Scorpio is capable of getting down and dirty. Sex is easiest between those Librans who are more relaxed, even a bit crude, and the more highly refined Scorpios. However, the differences in personality and approach to almost every aspect of daily life still make it hard for these two to relate.

If Libra will confront problems more directly and if Scorpio will avoid prodding or nagging, if Libra lets down all guards and allows Scorpio to devour him, this couple has a better chance for success long term.

SUMMARY

Scorpio is drawn to Libra's handsome features and charm. Libra is turned on by Scorpio's macho magnetism. In the bedroom, Libra likes most anything, though not always anal sex, which is a big part of sexual gratification for Scorpio. Scorpio has an opinion about everything and is committed to it. Although Libra is not naturally confrontational, he does love a good debate. Something about Scorpio's nature seems to trigger Libra, who then argues with Scorpio, no matter what the subject. If these two guys enjoy using sex to make up after "heated discussions," the sex will be pretty damn hot.

Libra ~ Sagittarius
The Scales and the Archer ~ perfect balance

This is a fun combination. Sagittarius and Libra share similar likes and dislikes, from traveling or camping, to gambling or spiritual retreats. They have a good time with sex and like to try it anywhere, on the beach, on the rooftops, certainly in the woods. They may also enjoy making videos of their lovemaking, as Sagittarius is a natural performer and Libra, a bit of an exhibitionist.

Libra, the Sign of commitment, understands that the best of relationships is between people who stand beside each other as partners, mutually independent. Libra is not looking for a mate to lean upon and will not tolerate someone who is clingy or demanding. In self-reliant Sagittarius, whose motto is "don't fence me in," Libra finds perfect balance.

The Archer is a dependable lover once ready for a long-term relationship, but nobody can rush him. Libra isn't pushy. Sagittarius is a social and outgoing man. He's frank, outspoken, charming, and witty. He does have a temper and can be secretive, but Libra has a knack for helping stressed out Sagittarius regain his normal affable demeanor.

Until Libra is ready for commitment, he can be very shallow in romance. After all Libra is ruled by Venus, the planet of beauty and physical love. Libra loves sex. Sagittarius, more passionate sexually, adds heat to Libra's calmer approach. With or without sex toys, within the range of mainstream sex or exploring outside its boundaries, they match each other well and have all it takes for a successful relationship.

SUMMARY

These two can share a delightful affair, be best friends, work together well, and have a lifelong intimate partnership. The only sticking point is timing. In other words, if Libra is still going through his fickle phase when Sagittarius is ready to settle down, Libra will cheat. Conversely, if Libra is ready for commitment, and Sagittarius is still playing the centaur stud, Libra will be heartbroken. For success long term, Sagittarius must remember to praise Libra and continue to romance him, or Libra will withhold sex. Sex can be a tool that Libra uses as a reward or punishment.

Libra ~ **Capricorn**
The Scales and the Goat ~ odd balance

Air Sign Libra and Earth Sign Capricorn might be expected to kick up more dust than to build anything solid, as they have trait after trait at odds with each other and yet the attraction is powerful. What brings them together?

The positives: reserved Capricorn is charmed by the warmth and effortless people skills of Libra. Libra is drawn to the quiet, courteous demeanor of Capricorn. Luxury-loving Libra appreciates the hard-driving goal orientation of Capricorn. Each is supportive of the other's ambitions. Both seek to avoid confrontation. Capricorn gets quiet and withdraws when there's discord. Libra backs away from arguments and tries to find a way to negotiate a compromise.

As to the differences, Libra is sociable while Capricorn is reserved. Libra is relaxed, impressionable, and a bit lazy. Capricorn is on guard, somewhat suspicious, and the hardest worker in the zodiac.

In bed, Capricorn likes to take it slow and easy but builds to considerable intensity and enjoys getting sweaty in the process. Libra appreciates a slow verbal buildup but not too long a session in the sheets and while sex will always be satisfying, Libra rarely breaks a sweat. Libra is generally rather mainstream in sexual behavior. There are some Capricorns who travel on the outer edge of sex. Put these two together and, in general, the affair is a brief one. A sexually moderate Capricorn and a somewhat experimental Libra will enjoy each other far more. Long term this relationship may work but will require ongoing effort.

SUMMARY

The division of responsibilities must be clearly defined. Libra will look for the easy way out and Capricorn isn't above using his manipulative skills to get what he wants. They share a desire to live well. For Libra life is dull and unsatisfying without at least a few luxuries, a dinner out, a cruise. Capricorn cares about what others think, so he wants a new car every couple of years. Both will work to fulfill these material desires. Flirtatious Libra will make Capricorn jealous even though the Goat loves seeing him charm the crowd. But all's well as long as Libra goes home exclusively with him.

Libra ~ Aquarius
The Scales and the Water Bearer ~ a delightful duo

The strongest elements of this relationship are friendship and social life. Libra and Aquarius have similar likes and dislikes, and even when they disagree, there is seldom much discord. They love to talk about everything, including sex. Sometimes their conversations are more exciting than the act itself. Sex may last five minutes but the discussion could carry them across a walking tour of Europe.

Aquarius wants sex daily. He's on a quest for deep emotional response. What he finds with Libra is more friendship than passion, but the quality of the communication and sense of companionship makes for a rewarding lifelong connection.

For both Signs, sexy words and images create the mood for sex. Reading erotic literature aloud is a major turn-on. Sexy videos are great, nothing crude, but rather those that are more erotic than pornographic. Dinner beside the river, or with a view of mountains, by a fireplace or in the woods is a sensual stimulus. The setting for sex is of greater importance to Libra than Aquarius, but for both, lighting matters, preferably not too bright, and the scent of vanilla is appealing.

In their sexual practices both Signs range from mainstream to experimental, including voyeurism, sex in public places, using food in sex play and for sex toys, primarily dildoes. Libra may have experienced more variety and will find Aquarius generally open to experimentation in such areas as the use of costumes, leather and latex, and some bondage. Bringing in the unexpected will add spark to their sex life.

SUMMARY

Libra is independent, doesn't necessarily want to run the show but will do what he wants to. Aquarius doesn't mind being led in some aspects of life. Where there's a disagreement, Libra might shy away from confrontation while Aquarius will face the issue head on without being argumentative. With two Air Signs like Libra and Aquarius, sex will be satisfying as both have similar sex drives, though there isn't likely to be the sustaining passion found with a Fire Sign, such as Aries, Leo, or Sagittarius. Sex may not move the earth but it will be frequent with a caring partner. A highly successful combination.

Libra ~ Pisces
The Scales and the Fish ~ mixed metaphor

Air Sign Libra mixed with Water Sign Pisces just goes flat. It starts out well. Pisces is idealistic, giving, gentle, refined, and devoted. Libra shares many of these traits, and at first they regard each other as being extremely similar. But they aren't. In fact, their personality differences give rise to general imbalance in the relationship. Pisces is a complex sign, not dominant but not about to be led either. Libra is a subtle Sign, and though independent, Libra doesn't like to take charge.

Libra's overall energy is very pleasant. He is genuinely nice. In a sustaining relationship and for exciting sex, he needs someone with raw energy. It is the Fire Signs who ignite his passion. A Water Sign like Pisces is fundamentally emotional and doesn't necessarily bring the spark of passion that Libra needs. Conversely, Pisces longs for a person who is decidedly earthy, very physical. Perhaps these two can be great friends, but in a sexual relationship, over time, they do not satisfy each other.

Sex in the early days will be wonderful. The romanticism of Pisces is exciting to Libra who enjoys seduction, candles, and incense to create the mood. For a while they have fun setting the stage, luxuriating in sensual pleasure, however, different things turn them on. Talking about sex off and on through the day is part of foreplay for Libra. With Pisces, foreplay begins in the bedroom. In the course of the relationship, while Pisces continues to desire romance, Libra is more satisfied simply fulfilling a sexual urge.

SUMMARY

This is a study in contrasts. Pisces wants a quiet homelife, steady and structured. Libra wants an active social life, mixing with a large circle of friends. Libra is a great support for someone else and wants a decisive partner. Pisces resists that role. Sometimes, someone has to take charge. It is hard for either man to make decisions that affect both. As co-workers and friends, these men relate well, but in an intimate relationship Pisces is too indirect for Libra, and Libra is too unwilling to confront problems to satisfy Pisces. In bed the same negatives may undermine the passion.

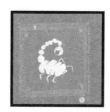

Scorpio ~ Scorpio
Two Scorpions together ~ passion or poison

Two Scorpios, both powerhouses, both passionate, both suspicious, and both jealous. They are inherently competitive. The sex is incredibly exciting. From the minute a sexual encounter begins, each Scorpio is out to impress the other with both duration and intensity.

They have the same likes and dislikes. Kissing gets things started, being taken by force or having the other do the initiating is a turn-on. They like taking time before going to the most erogenous zone, building up fairly quickly but with control and coming to a simultaneous earth-moving orgasm.

Scorpios react to each other the way magnets do, either pulled together or pushed apart. The attraction is instantaneous and breathtaking or both parties warily keep a careful distance. Even their body language makes this apparent. They face each other openly or lower their heads and keep their arms wrapped across their chests.

There is no balance with two like Signs together. Rather there is a doubling up of all the characteristics, good and bad, that each Sign possesses. Scorpio is both secretive and on a deep level, somewhat insecure. Seemingly without provocation one Scorpio may turn on the other issuing accusations that come from unresolved or even unfounded suspicions. Should these two get into an angry debate or suffer an ugly breakup, the grudge is likely to continue through the rest of time.

If there is ever to be any peace on the planet for two Scorpios, it is crucial that each be totally open with the other.

SUMMARY

Scorpio is a compulsive Sign. When he puts his mind to something, he's relentless in its pursuit. Once he lays eyes on the object of his affection he will not be deterred until that man is in his bed. The sex is intense, the intimacy extraordinary, and while they are in the bedroom they get along famously. What works against them comes out of the fundamental negative qualities of Scorpio—obstinacy, jealousy, and anger. Scorpio hates to have those feelings triggered, but invariably one will make the other jealous, rage will be ignited, and the relationship will go up in flames.

Scorpio ~ **Sagittarius**
The Scorpion and the Archer ~ don't worry be happy

This is a difficult pairing but one with potential. Sagittarius, the zodiac's philosopher, says, "the goal of life is happiness." Scorpio doesn't understand that idea. When life is going well, Scorpio is waiting for the other shoe to drop. When life is tough, Scorpio is calm, confident, and ready to take action. Sagittarius is certainly up to life's challenge but feels quite content when life is good. Sagittarius's optimism brightens Scorpio. Scorpio's quiet depth comforts Sagittarius.

In bed, add Scorpio's passion to Sagittarius's endurance and one gets steamy sex, perhaps not overly varied, but passionate and satisfying. Their pleasures are parallel, including the occasional use of sex toys and having sex in out-of-the-ordinary locations. They also enjoy participating in a ménage à trois and exhibitionism in gay-friendly areas.

When Scorpio wants to achieve something, the approach is like a laser beam, moving straight ahead, unswerving, to accomplish that goal. Sagittarius prefers a broad overview before choosing a course of action. He wants to see the entire forest. Scorpio can be put off by what he views as a cursory overview. Sagittarius believes Scorpio takes too narrow a view.

Sagittarius is famous for letting fly words that cut like an arrow. Though powerful, Scorpio is also a highly emotional, easily wounded Water Sign with a remarkable memory. Those words leave indelible scars. For the relationship to succeed, maturity is needed. Scorpio must back off from competition and enjoy the ardent nature of Sagittarius. Sagittarius needs to beware of shooting from the hip.

SUMMARY

This relationship can be successful long term with some effort. Both enjoy a range of activities, including spending time with friends and family, traveling, and perhaps gambling. They are ardent lovers matching each other well in sexual likes, dislikes, and frequency. It is necessary for Sagittarius to come to terms with Scorpio's secretive nature and not take it personally. This is difficult for Sagittarius, as he easily sizes up other people but can't read Scorpio. Scorpio needs to curb his possessive nature, as Sagittarius is a freedom-loving Sign. Conversely, Sagittarius has to be clear about his commitment to Scorpio.

Scorpio ~ **Capricorn**
The Scorpion and the Goat ~ the perfect pair

Ideal balance. Scorpio represents the power of desire and has a great need for accomplishment, Capricorn is motivated to achieve, ambitious, and the hardest worker in the zodiac. When Capricorn needs to make a decision, the Goat keeps the subject closely guarded, telling nobody what ideas or plans are on tap until quite certain of a course or direction. That behavior might be disconcerting to some but not to Scorpio who is secretive by nature. Scorpio is far more emotional than Capricorn, and that softens what appears to be an overly pragmatic approach to life that Capricorn projects.

There are few differences between these two, but one is important. Capricorn cares enormously what other people think and Scorpio simply doesn't. If Capricorn has enough money to paint either the inside or outside of the house, Capricorn paints the outside. Conversely, Scorpio would paint the inside.

The physical relationship is satisfying, as these two are similar in almost all aspects of sexuality. They like the same sex acts, the same frequency and forcefulness. Amount of time spent in a sexual encounter is of little importance to either Sign. Both are experimental and Capricorn will match Scorpio fetish for fetish from bondage to ménage à trois all the way to orgies and in some cases, sado-masochism.

While Scorpio's possessiveness turns off several other Signs, Capricorn finds it reassuring and feels secure. Some might find Capricorn impersonal, but Scorpio is comfortable knowing there is ample compensation in the richness of their sex life.

SUMMARY

Hot and heavy in the bedroom, sex in many flavors, well past vanilla, both enjoy the escapism of fantasy in their sex lives. They are natural partners in all other regards. Both strive to succeed financially, Scorpio so he can do what he wants, Capricorn so he'll be respected in the community. Both are fairly private about being gay. Scorpio because it's his nature to be secretive. Capricorn because of his deep desire to be successful in the business world is cautious about being too "out." Privately, when Capricorn relaxes his guard, the relationship in and out of bed is fulfilling.

Scorpio ~ Aquarius
The Scorpion and the Water Bearer ~ conflicting species

"I say potato and you say patahto. I say tomato and you say tomahto," sums it up. These two just don't speak the same language. Exceptions may exist, but generally Scorpio and Aquarius make as difficult a relationship as any two people are likely to form. In love affairs, after a while, they annoy each other.

Neither Sign is even likely to find the other sexually attractive. When they do, the first few encounters will be intense but the passion is unlikely to last. Aquarius seeks sensation through sex, trying a variety of approaches, but from an intellectual core. Scorpio is all about getting down, dirty, and sweaty.

When Scorpio is after something, the objective is the only focus. Scorpio aims straight ahead, stripping away all that is superfluous to attain that end. To Aquarius this is very limiting. Aquarius, after that same objective, sees ten new elements to enrich the goal and must, therefore, take a very different and circuitous path. Scorpio finds this maddening. When Scorpio wants comforting. Aquarius offers levelheaded advice. When in an emotional state the last thing on earth Scorpio wants is calm advice. And when Aquarius is distressed, getting an emotional response from Scorpio only makes matters worse.

For Aquarius, seduction is word play. For Scorpio, it's "Let's get to the point." For Aquarius, the sexiest part of the body is the brain. For Scorpio, it is smack dab between his legs. A long-distance relationship may be the most satisfying long-term romance for this unlikely twosome.

SUMMARY

They meet at a party. Aquarius knows everyone in the room and everyone likes him. He's a great conversationalist, at ease talking about a broad spectrum of subjects. Scorpio is entranced. Aquarius keeps the conversation going and going, even when the two have arrived at Scorpio's place and Scorpio is shedding his clothes and propelling Aquarius to the bed. Aquarius is electrified by Scorpio's passion but over time can't match it. He's turned off by Scorpio's possessiveness and need to dominate. Scorpio isn't satisfied with Aquarius's cool intellectual response, wanting something more earthy and emotional. Not a formula for contentment.

Scorpio ~ Pisces
The Scorpion and the Fish ~ happy surf and turf

This is a great combination in friendship, business, or sexual relationships. They share similar values and pleasures, cherishing family and enjoying the comfort and quiet of their home. They love to cuddle aside from sex but also need privacy and periods of retreat. Pisces has periods of self-pity. Scorpio provides strength and comfort. Sometimes Scorpio has a hard time opening up, but Pisces has an uncanny ability to understand what's going on inside the secretive Scorpion. All their communications have an ESP quality, going beyond words. This empathy extends to the bedroom.

These two can spend a week having sex without surfacing for anything beyond room service. Scorpio believes that nobody is his equal at lovemaking. In Pisces he has met his match. Pisces has super endurance and never gets burned out. Sexually, these two passionate Signs enjoy almost anything, anywhere, and anytime. Their timing is in sync and they frequently achieve orgasm simultaneously.

One difference between them is that Scorpio exudes a kind of energy force field, seen by all as extremely strong, whereas Pisces, not an aggressive Sign, may seem to be weak. Surprise! Surprise! Pisces has a remarkable ability, perhaps it's hypnosis, to convince people to his opinion.

Scorpio and Pisces are both sensitive, emotional, and empathetic Water Signs. Being near the water, from the ocean to a lake or a stream helps them to get back in touch with themselves and each other. This is a relationship that should prove gratifying forever, in life and in love.

SUMMARY

They make great friends and great lovers, sharing sexual likes and dislikes. Sensitive to each other, matched in passion and endurance, this couple could happily grow old together. They'll enjoy the same music, movies, and food. They'll be happy whether they can take Caribbean cruises or merely go for walks on the beach, depending on the size of their bank accounts. Scorpio should make no mistake about it, Pisces is every bit as powerful as he is. The style differs, not the substance. This is a fifty/fifty partnership, and that is both gratifying and unusual for the normally dominant Scorpio.

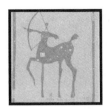

Sagittarius ~ Sagittarius
Two Archers together ~ cupid's arrow or poison dart?

They're so busy, their minds are everywhere but where they should be to really get involved with one another. They have disagreements, but Sagittarius loves a good debate. Sagittarius is impulsive and may come home from work on Friday to say, " Pack your bags, we're heading for the mountains." Speaking of mountains, Sagittarius tends to see the big picture, the forest, overlooking the details, like the trees. In this relationship someone has to pay attention to mundane, daily reality.

Sagittarius is both the Sign of the gambler, a risk taker, and the philosopher who knows the goal of life is happiness. Since Jupiter, the planet of abundance, rules Sagittarius, most of the time they're lucky. In all, Sagittarius is a laid back, mellow personality, willing to take chances, hard to pin down, won't be dictated to by others, and does not tell others how to live their lives.

One admits to being jealous, the other says he is not. One believes in monogamy, the other will strive for it but would enjoy an open relationship were it possible. Neither is overly concerned about the setting for sex, enjoying sex in varied locations, such as the woods or the beach. And yet, the sex is best when one bothers to set the stage by lighting candles and incense or playing music quietly in the background. The fulfillment of the sex may not be wonderful, but the enjoyment that each finds with the total personality of another Sagittarius will be great.

SUMMARY

They can talk up a blue streak about anything and love a good debate. Topics of interest range from religion and spirituality to local politics and world government. The heat of their debates will dwarf any heat of passion in the bedroom. In fact the sex may be less than thrilling because both want to be the center of attention. In a relationship, what's good is that each understands that the other needs to feel free and unencumbered. After all, "Don't fence me in" is Sagittarius's theme song. A fling or a ménage à trois might be just the thing to keep their relationship lively.

Sagittarius ~ Capricorn
The Archer and the Goat ~ a worthwhile challenge

This is a great combination. Both are sincere and dependable. They balance each other. Capricorn is inspired by the imagination of Sagittarius. Since Capricorn can be overly pragmatic, they're apt to lose touch with their own creativity. Dreamer Sagittarius looks at the sky and in the clouds sees castles and dragons. Capricorn says, "It looks like rain."

Capricorn is cautious. Sagittarius is spontaneous, apt to wake up on a Saturday morning and say, "I feel like getting out of town. Pack your bags. Let's go." Capricorn asks, "Where are we going? How long will it take to get there? Where are we staying? How much will it cost?"

In the bedroom, Sagittarius strives to excite Capricorn with busy hands, oral sex, and wonderful body moves. Capricorn's responsiveness stimulates Sagittarius to be more inventive, and that's something the Archer finds rewarding. Sexually, Capricorn runs the gamut from mainstream to very experimental. Sagittarius is an experimental lover, so sex with mainstream Capricorn won't be quite as satisfactory. But those Capricorns who enjoy a wider range of sexual practices, perhaps including bondage and S&M, may find a very willing partner in the Archer.

There are a few areas of potential trouble. Sagittarius, the gambler of the zodiac, less than cautious with money, may cause frugal Capricorn stress. Ambitious Capricorn is apt to be disconcerted by Sagittarius's laid-back attitude. Where Sagittarius may be blunt, Capricorn will be diplomatic. But both are goodhearted and strive to meet the needs of the other.

SUMMARY

A Capricorn man always looks appropriate. He carries himself well and even when most casually dressed, he somehow gives the impression that he's wearing a three-piece suit. Sagittarius finds this decidedly attractive. Conversely, Capricorn is drawn to the Archer's casual self-confidence. Conversation is lively, even contentious but stimulating. Capricorn thinks deeply and Sagittarius takes a broad view. Their friendship is rewarding and their sex life exciting. Still their differences need attention. Capricorn is a bit staid and needs to plan everything with care. Sagittarius is freewheeling and spontaneous. It will take patience and willingness to yield to keep this couple happy long term.

Sagittarius ~ Aquarius
The Archer and the Water Bearer ~ as good as it gets

This is the perfect, happy couple. Where they go is always exciting whether it's a Cape Cod bed and breakfast or a ski-lodge in Aspen. They always have the best sex when they get away from it all. Then Sagittarius turns full attention to sex and won't be distracted and Aquarius, too, will focus on the business at hand, which is pleasure.

Sagittarius is a Fire Sign. Aquarius is an Air Sign. These two elements are always compatible, as friends, in business, and in love affairs. Neither Sign triggers any insecurity in the other. Sagittarius needs freedom and Aquarius is not possessive. Both enjoy a wide range of activities that might include traveling, sports, the arts, and charitable functions.

The Archer and the Water Bearer are truly made for each other. While Aquarius has a less than lustrous reputation sexually, Sagittarius has the ability to heat things up. For Aquarius, not only initial excitement but also all through the sexual experience, words are the primary stimulus and Sagittarius can tell a wonderful story. In fact, Sagittarius will turn Aquarius on as much by talking about sex as with kisses or sensual touching.

Sagittarius is somewhat experimental in his approach to sex, enjoying sex outdoors and some bondage or role-playing. The Archer isn't overly interested in sex toys or sexual behaviors such as S&M. Sagittarius may enjoy long sessions of sex on occasion, but most of the time prefers to get to the heart of the matter fairly quickly. All this suits Aquarius perfectly.

SUMMARY

The attraction is immediate. The friendship is fulfilling. Aquarius is thrilled with Sagittarius's physique and the size of his penis. Sagittarius is turned on by the Aquarian's enthusiasm and excitement about life in general. When they first meet, Sagittarius picks up a sense of electricity from Aquarius. Sex will be intense. The build-up verbally will take longer than the act itself. To maintain this initial excitement Aquarius will want to bring variety into the bedroom. These two may very well have a relationship that lasts lifelong as they satisfy each other on all levels, emotional, sexual, and spiritual.

Sagittarius ~ Pisces
The Archer and the Fish ~ an uphill challenge

The war, the conflict, is non-stop. For Sagittarius, loving a good debate, the comparison of philosophies is stimulating and Sagittarius is curious about Pisces's ideas, but sometimes Sagittarius finds Pisces petty. This is a tough combination for long-term relationships. Both in bed and out, this combination comes down to being an experiment.

There are some areas of compatibility. Both are thoughtful and spiritual though Sagittarius is more religious in a traditional sense and Pisces is more open to New Age ideas. Sagittarius is the philosopher, seeking balance between freedom and responsibility, seeking happiness. Pisces is the Sign of sacrifice and service, seeking spiritual fulfillment.

The differences are vast. Pisces is sensitive and refined, Sagittarius is blunt, rash, and at least in speech, capable of crudeness. Pisces can be hard to pin down. As the twelfth Sign of the zodiac, Pisces possesses some characteristics of all the Signs. It is also a dual Sign, two fishes swimming in opposite directions, suggesting Pisces's complexities. Sagittarius is sincere, honest to a fault, independent, and upbeat. Sagittarius has a remarkable ability for shrugging things off. Pisces wallows in problems for a bit and is given to self-pity.

Both are passionate lovers. Initially the sex will be extraordinary. It is all the other aspects of this relationship—the practical realities and philosophical differences—that prove destructive. After a while, even in bed, fiery Sagittarius and watery Pisces produce more fizzle than sizzle. Pisces wants far more romance and drama, while Sagittarius wants more energetic expressions of passion.

SUMMARY

An ideal date or evening out for Sagittarius might be kayaking or going to the putting range. For Pisces it's dinner at home or at a quiet restaurant surrounded by soft lighting and romantic music. When Pisces travels he wants to visit his homeland or historic sites such as Pompeii, Athens, or Jerusalem. Sagittarius prefers the track at Saratoga, Monte Carlo, or Las Vegas. Sagittarius gambles and if he loses, worries about the mortgage later. This drives Pisces to distraction. In short time Sagittarius will wander and Pisces will seek the comforting arms of some tall, handsome stranger.

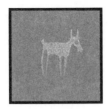

Capricorn ~ **Capricorn**
Two Goats ~ no head butting, just contentment

Contented in public and private, they go out looking terrific and turn heads. In bed this relationship is dynamic because each wants to impress the other. The sex is long, easy, and enjoyable.

Capricorn finds one classic style of dress and sticks with it, one hairstyle worn for decades, one favorite path to walk through the park. Stability and constancy are the earmarks of this Sign. Sound boring? It's not. Capricorn knows how to simplify trivialities, leaving time for the important aspects of life.

These wise Goats are willing to delay and deny pleasure until significant goals have been accomplished. Their pride requires that they be seen as upstanding members of the community. In fact, they care enormously about what the neighbors will say. With similar values and commitment to take the proper steps to achieve them, two Capricorns have solid mutual respect.

Capricorn, the hardest worker in the zodiac, is indefatigable and exceptionally persistent. These qualities, in the bedroom, make Capricorn an excellent lover. The Goat does not take sex lightly. Behind closed doors, Capricorn's reticence dissolves, passion is released. Sex is usually slow and drawn out, showing this Sun Sign's qualities of endurance and persistence. Capricorn is a lover with a mission, to achieve and accomplish a partner's pleasure and their own.

While most Capricorns enjoy primarily conventional sex, there is a good-sized group within this Sun Sign that loves more varied sex play. They are turned on by bondage, dominance and submission, and in some cases by sadomasochism.

SUMMARY

They may not feel an instant chemistry upon encountering each another, as the attraction is more intellectual than physical. There is a sense of reflection. They share similar tastes in food, clothes, furnishings, and architectural styles, have compatible ideas and philosophies. In a relationship, Capricorn wants commitment, although that may not require sexual exclusivity. Having an occasional other sex partner either for a ménage à trois or as a side order may not be a deal breaker for these two. Sex will rarely be brief and always satisfying. Two Goats form a comfortable, secure, and thoroughly pleasurable life together in bed and out.

Capricorn ~ Aquarius
The Goat and the Water Bearer ~ interest or irritation

Though the attraction may be powerful, this is a difficult connection in the bedroom and in all aspects of the relationship. Capricorn is practical and cautious, whereas Aquarius seems so open and full of inspiration. It looks easy for Aquarius to enter a crowd and talk with people. Capricorn is more guarded.

Initially Aquarius finds comfort in that wonderful Capricorn sense of grounding and stability. Later, this same quality seems stifling. For Capricorn there is frustration trying to feel closer, more connected. Aquarius remains somehow distant.

When these two get into conversation, though they may have very different opinions, the interaction is stimulating. One stimulus leads to another, and what is truly a developing friendship appears to be a fledgling romance.

Once they tumble onto a bed, a couch, or any other suitable site, their differences become glaringly apparent. Capricorn, like all Earth Signs, enjoys physicality in all forms. Sex is a release from the confines of proper behavior. Aquarius is more turned on by words, by erotica, than by the messy, sweaty sex that is more to Capricorn's liking. For sex to work, Capricorn must set the stage verbally to excite Aquarius, and Aquarius has to talk less and do more to satisfy Capricorn.

Capricorn wants to plan ahead and make a date for sex and likes to repeat the same performance. If it worked once why change it? "If it ain't broke, why fix it?" Aquarius gets bored. Short term there will be interest and excitement. Long term, irritation.

SUMMARY

Their conversations will be dynamic, stimulating, and wide ranging in subject matter, but their differences in sex drive, attitude towards sex, and nature of sexual pleasure will make sustaining a relationship difficult. Aquarius is an iconoclast, wanting to change things. Capricorn wants to sustain the status quo. Capricorn is possessive, Aquarius flirtatious. Sexually, Aquarius wants to try everything that is new and different. Capricorn likes the tried and true. The exception to the rule is the more experimental Capricorn who does match up quite well with Aquarius, for example, sharing a liking for sexual threesomes and perhaps water sports.

Capricorn ~ Pisces
The Goat and the Fish ~ contented species

Capricorn and Pisces are highly compatible Signs that relate to each other comfortably in all types of relationships from friendship to business to romance. They are inherently in sync with one another and find it comfortable discussing most topics without friction. They have the potential to be an enviably happy couple.

The pragmatism of Capricorn is balanced by the idealism of Pisces. Capricorn is cautious, Pisces is giving. Capricorn takes stock of situations and people, observing behavior in order to understand circumstances, while impressionable Pisces uses intuition to achieve the same understanding. Pisces is a more social Sign than Capricorn helping ease any of Capricorn's reservations when dealing with groups of people. Capricorn is the stabilizing energy when Pisces's fancies grow a bit wild.

In matters sexual, both Signs are noted for their endurance. They prefer to be unhurried, enjoying touching, kissing, and oral sex, perhaps leading to multiple orgasms over a fairly lengthy stretch of time. They understand each other in bed with little guidance needed from one to the other to obtain maximum pleasure. The difference in their sexual expression has to do with the importance of romance and a sense of stage set that is so vital for Pisces. Most of the time Capricorn couldn't care less about the environment as long as it is clean. Pisces, on the other hand, wants a setting that gives rise to fantasies. Candles, incense, silky draperies or satin sheets, and messages of love make Pisces all the more excited.

SUMMARY

Capricorn is aware of his own sexual powers, maybe even his perversions. Pisces brings out his tenderness, the inner softie that's buttoned up inside that three-piece suit. Both men are highly flirtatious, sometimes jealous and possessive. They can talk to each other about most everything and work through such problems, strengthening their relationship and achieving trust. In matters sexual, both are highly experimental and enjoy exploring a range of sexual activities including bondage, domination, and the use of various sex toys. Combining their capacity to resolve conflict and their inherent sexual harmony suggests a relationship that can last through time.

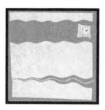

Aquarius ~ Aquarius
Two Water Bearers ~ stimulate the mind, sex follows

This is the buddy relationship. "You do your thing and I'll do mine." Both are independent people and while apt to find one job, one house, one model car, and stay with each forever, Aquarius will not tolerate feeling possessed in a relationship.

They love to discuss their activities. When Aquarians talk about the things they feel passionately, from politics to music, careers to cars, that passion spills over into sexual energy. For Air Sign Aquarius, conversation stimulates the mind and the Water Bearer says the most important sex organ is the brain.

More than the physical, features or body type, more than chemistry, it's ideas that turn on sexual excitement for Aquarius. Erotic literature and talking dirty are both sure turn-ons. While pornographic videos may be stimulating when he masturbates, porn is dependent upon images more than words, so it isn't the turn-on of choice when he's with a partner.

There are times that words aren't the best way to reach each other, emotional times, when a touch or a hug goes a lot further than words. That is when Aquarians need to put aside the cool, calm, collected behavior, get in touch with feelings, and demonstrate affection directly.

As these two make very good friends and share all basic likes and dislikes, they may well be able to make a lifelong relationship work. Sex will not be the most important part of their union and will require role-playing or various accouterments to keep lively, but it can prove satisfying.

SUMMARY

Truth is, they've had better sex elsewhere. Sex isn't that important to Aquarius. Sure orgasm feels great, but they're much more interested in being out and about, meeting new people and finding out who's doing whom. Face it, Aquarius needs stimulus. The best way to handle this is directly. Admit out loud the need for extracurricular encounters and head out to the scene. Competition will be an occasional problem, but Aquarius is skilled at cooperation and can find solutions to problems, thus enabling their relationship to continue even through hard times. What's wrong with a lifelong commitment based on a true meeting of the minds?

Aquarius ~ Pisces
The Water Bearer and the Fish ~
more friction than fun and games

This is a rare and uncomfortable combination. Aquarius is rational where Pisces is intuitive. Aquarius confronts situations. Pisces recedes from them. Aquarius is cool and diplomatic, detached and impersonal. Aquarius enjoys being in public but is uncomfortable with intimacy. Pisces is emotional, creates very intense friendships, is romantic, sentimental, and enjoys nostalgia. In fact, Pisces has a strong need to stay connected to the past, whereas Aquarius is involved with the future. Pisces is the personality who belongs to the historical society or the preservation commission. Aquarius serves on the community planning board.

When it comes to sex, talking dirty and reading excerpts from erotic literature turns Aquarius on. This is new and different to Pisces who will respond, for a while. Pisces wants romance and a stage set for sex. The environment is of little matter to Aquarius. Yes, the passion of Pisces turns Aquarius on in the beginning, but over time, Aquarius gets bored with the long sessions Pisces so loves. In addition, the aloofness of Aquarius triggers feelings of uncertainty in Pisces. Then Pisces gets clingy, which will never work with independent Aquarius.

For more than a passing fling, Aquarius has to talk less and romance more, with mood setting items like wine and roses, music and candles, and Pisces needs to stimulate that wonderful Aquarius brain with conversation. Best advice for would-be Aquarius/Pisces couples: have a long enough courtship, at least two years, to be sure this is what you want before holding the commitment ceremony.

SUMMARY

Each finds the other's idiosyncrasies terribly unsettling. In a relationship Pisces wants a feeling of security and commitment, "We two against the world." What Aquarius wants is someone to come home to when he feels like coming home. The independence of Aquarius triggers the vulnerability of Pisces. Out on the scene, Pisces is a terrible flirt and while he may not mean anything by it, Aquarius dislikes such behavior. Aquarius may not often be flirtatious, but when he is, Pisces hates it. Aquarius doesn't fulfill Pisces sexual needs. Simply put, Aquarius wants variety to stimulate sexual excitement while Pisces wants romance.

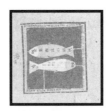

Pisces ~ Pisces
Two Fish ~ swimming happily round and round

Pisces is an idealistic, sensitive, and refined Sign. It rules medicine and healing, and many Pisces work with sick and needy people. These fields require strength, the strength of compassion, not aggression.

Pisceans manage to achieve their objectives by a sort of maneuvering more akin to hypnosis than to overt assertive behavior. Pisces is not known for being particularly direct in confronting difficulties. This is a problem in all their relationships, particularly between two Pisces.

Because Pisces so wish to avoid confrontation, they may concede in a discussion, seeming to concur and then go off and do whatever they want to do. This is not a successful way to conduct a partnership. Simply put, Pisces needs to learn to state "I understand your position. I don't agree with you."

In a new relationship, two Pisces are like happy flower children, out there making love, not war, following the music wherever it may take them, and in the bedroom life is great. They want to have sex virtually every day and enjoy a range of experimental sexual activities at a leisurely, romantic pace.

What is necessary to insure that Pisces will make a relationship last long term is a division of labor. Someone has to get out of bed, out of the house, and be practical. Someone has to deal with the down and dirty every day mundane realities. Neither wants to. Each tries to maneuver the other into doing it. Solve this problem and these two Fish can swim successfully side by side.

SUMMARY

Each uses the same ploys and practices to achieve his objective. When Pisces wants something that the other disagrees about, he puts up a brave front demanding it. But Pisces #2 knows full well that the straightness of posture and strength of his words isn't backed up by any potential physical aggression. Pisces #1 says, "I want to do it this way." Pisces #2 says, "No." And that's the end of it. One might get angry or just laugh it off. Laughing it off is for the best. After all, he truly is the best sex ever. Why blow it?

Secrets to Great Sex Questionnaire

Part 1: Background Information

Date of birth: _____ Time of birth: _____

City and State of birth: _____

Male/Female: _____ Gay/Straight/Bisexual: _____

Marital status: _____

How often do you think about sex? (Daily, weekly, preoccupied with it, seldom)

_____

How much time do you like to spend having sex? (One hour, half hour, more, less)
How much of that is foreplay?

_____

Do you enjoy quickies? _____

Are you sexually in the mainstream, more experimental, or open to anything?

_____

How often per week do you masturbate?

_____

What's your attitude toward casual sex? (Love it, it's fine, it's immoral, it's unsafe, other)

_____

_____

Do you believe in monogamy? Why?

_____

_____

Does sex have a spiritual significance for you? How so?

_____

_____

_____

What's your attitude toward pornography? (Love it, hate it, no interest)

_____

_____

Part 2: Attraction

What attracts you to someone? What turns you on? (Please specify physical characteristics, specific behaviors, attitudes, etc.)

_____

_____

_____

What might turn you off?

_____

_____

_____

Are you flirtatious and, if so, how much?

_____

_____

_____

Are you jealous?

_____

_____

_____

Part 3: Developing the Relationship

What do you enjoy doing on a date?

_____

_____

_____

How much cuddling do you enjoy, aside from sex?

_____

_____

_____

How do you demonstrate affection for your partner? (Specific acts of kindness)

_____

_____

_____

_____

How do you feel about public displays of affection?

_____

_____

_____

How long do you want to know someone before getting sexual?

_____

_____

Part 4: Foreplay

Are you comfortable initiating sexual activities?

_____

_____

_____

What puts you in the mood for sex? (Favorite music, nature of the environment, kind of food, aromas, activities such as eating, showering, watching porn videos, other)

_____

_____

_____

Part 5: Having Sex

Where do you like to have sex?

_____

_____

_____

_____

How important is the sexual environment to you? (Cleanliness, orderliness, lighting, décor, etc.)

_____

_____

_____

_____

What time of day do you prefer to have sex?

_____

_____

_____

How tactile are you? Do you like to run your hands over your lover's body? (A lot, a little)

_____

_____

How oral are you? (How much do you enjoy deep kissing on the mouth, kissing your lover's body, oral sex, rimming, other)

_____

_____

How do you communicate to your partner your wants and needs, by words or gestures or both?

_____

_____

What sex acts do you like most? (Kissing, oral sex, anal sex, mutual masturbation, fondling breasts, other)

_____

_____

What sex acts do you like least?

_____

_____

Are you vocal during sex? A lot or a little?

_____

How do you reach an orgasm? (Oral sex, masturbation, combination, anal sex)

_____

How often do you reach orgasm? (All the time, often, seldom)

_____

Some people are very concerned about bringing their partner to climax before having an orgasm themselves. Others strive to reach orgasm together. Which is true for you?

_____

What's the best position for you to achieve orgasm? (Being on top, doggie style, spooning [stomach to back], facing side by side, sixty-nine)

_____

_____

For some people the taste of their partner's cum or secretions is unpleasant. If that's true for you, what do you do about the taste?

_____

_____

How do you handle his cum? (Swallow, rub it on yourself, other)

_____

_____

How often per week do you want to have sex?

_____

After sex what do you like to do? (Go out together, shower, sleep, take a walk, etc.)

_____

_____

Part 6: Intimacy

Do you enjoy watching your partner during sex and orgasm?

_____

_____

Do you enjoy being watched?

_____

_____

_____

What smells on your partner do you enjoy? (Skin, particular body parts, colognes, other)

_____

_____

What tastes on your partner do you enjoy?

_____

_____

Part 7: Fantasies and Fetishes

All people experience sex fantasies; we use them to arouse ourselves for self-pleasure and with a partner. Describe your sex fantasies.

_____

_____

_____

_____

As a lover, what's your best skill? (How you use your hands, tongue, body, other)

_____

_____

_____

Describe a wonderful sexual encounter—romantic or aggressive—complete with sights, smells, sounds, and location that made it extraordinary for you.

_____

_____

_____

_____

_____

_____

_____

Check off the fetishes/toys/behaviors you've tried:

__ Using sex toys (dildos, vibrators, body clips, etc. . . . Please specify)

_____

__ Anal (giving)	__ Anal (receiving)	__ Bondage
__ Chains	__ Cross-dressing	__ Dominance & Submission
__ Electricity	__ Enemas	__ Exhibitionism
__ Feet	__ Fisting (giving)	__ Fisting (receiving)
__ Hairy	__ Hot wax/ice cubes	__ Interracial
__ Leather and Latex	__ Long fingernails	__ Ménage à trois
__ Orgies	__ Piercings	__ Sadomasochism
__ Sex in public places	__ Shaved	__ Shoes and boots
__ Spanking	__ Tattoos	__ Underwear
__ Uniforms	__ Using food	__ Voyeurism
__ Water sports	__ Wearing costumes	
__ Other (specify)		

_____

THANK YOU FOR ANSWERING THIS QUESTIONNAIRE

Glossary of Terms

Air Signs: Gemini, Libra, and Aquarius. These are Signs of communication, the intellect. They filter life through their minds.

Anal sex: having intercourse or using sex toys in the anus

Body clips: also called clamps, sex toys that pinch flesh; used on nipples, genitals, and other body parts

Bondage: any act that incorporates restraints placed on the body to limit movement

Candaulism: sex act in which two people engage in sex and the third party watches

Chains: a form of restraint used in bondage or domination

Cross-dressing: wearing clothes of the opposite gender

Deprivation: *See* Sensory deprivation.

Dominance & Submission: consensual role-playing in which one partner allows the other to have control over his or her behavior

Earth Signs: Taurus, Virgo, and Capricorn. These are the practical Signs. They function best handling the day-to-day business of life.

Electricity: use of electrical devices as a sexual stimulation

Exhibitionism: performing sexual acts in public places for the thrill of being watched

Experimental: A range of sexual behaviors that goes beyond the mainstream actions of kissing, oral sex, and intercourse. These may include such behaviors as anal sex, use of sex toys that might include various dildoes, vibrators, and anal plugs, wearing costumes or uniforms, having sex in public places, light bondage, and dominance and submission.

Fetish: a sexual fascination involving a particular body part or object

Fire Signs: Aries, Leo, and Sagittarius. These are Signs of action and inspiration. They filter life through the ability to solve problems and get things done.

Fisting: insertion of the hand into the anus

Foot Fetish: fascination with feet or shoes

Frottage: often referred to as dry humping, rubbing against another person to attain sexual gratification

Hot wax: dripping candle wax onto flesh

Interracial: sexual preference for a partner of a race other than one's own

Long fingernails: fingernails, extended naturally or artificially, that provide sexual stimulus

Mainstream: range of sexuality including cuddling, kissing, fondling, oral sex, intercourse, and the use of sex toys such as dildoes and vibrators

Men/women in uniform: enjoying sex with people in costumes—usually people in positions of authority, such as a police officer, fireman, or member of the armed services

Ménage à trois: sex with two partners simultaneously

Open sexual practices: willing to try most sex acts, which might include sadomasochism, water sports, and fisting and the use of toys such as gags, cock and ball torture, sounds, electric stimulation, ropes, whips and paddles, and body clips

Orgies: participating in sex in a group of four or more people

Piercings: inserting needles into the skin to enhance sexual pleasure or to add body jewelry

Rimming: a part of anal play, using the tongue to lick and stimulate the partner's anus

Sadomasochism: The consensual use of pain and humiliation in sexual play. SM usually includes bondage, dominance and submission, and spanking.

Sensory deprivation: an attempt to eliminate any or all of the five senses

Sex in public places: having sex in places outside the bedroom, such as in cars, on beaches, in public bathrooms

Shoes or boots: using footwear to enhance sexual excitement

Sounds: a medical device; a metal rod inserted into the urethra to stimulate the prostate

Spanking: form of discipline used in dominance and submission play, varieties of meaning are achieved by the costumes included in the play

Sun Signs:

Aries Fire Sign, represents people born
between March 21 and April 19

Taurus Earth Sign, represents people born
between April 20 and May 20

Gemini Air Sign, represents people born
between May 21 and June 20

Cancer Water Sign, represents people born
between June 21 and July 22

Leo Fire Sign, represents people born
between July 23 and August 22

Virgo Earth Sign, represents people born
between August 23 and September 22

Libra Air Sign, represents people born
between September 23 and October 22

Scorpio Water Sign, represents people born
between October 23 and November 21

Sagittarius Fire Sign, represents people born
between November 22 and December 21

Capricorn Earth Sign, represents people born
between December 22 and January 19

Aquarius Air Sign, represents people born
between January 20 and February 18

Pisces Water Sign, represents people born
between February 19 and March 20

Tattoos: Injecting indelible dyes into the skin; the process of being tattooed is sexually exciting to some people.

Tantric sex: method of extending sexual arousal with use of meditation and breathing techniques

Using food: incorporating edible substances into the act of sex

Voyeurism: watching other people engage in sex

Water Signs: Cancer, Scorpio, and Pisces. These are the intuitive Signs. They filter life through their emotions.

Water sports: or golden showers; sex play involving urine

Wearing costumes: sexual role-playing in which a partner wears garments, such as French maid, schoolgirl, cowgirl, cowboy, pony outfit, etc.

Wearing leather or latex: using costumes made of leather or latex that fit the body tightly

About the Author

Myrna Lamb is a professional astrologer, with thirty years experience in the field, and a radio personality. On the air, Myrna hosted a variety of call-in programs, first on astrology, then a general advice show, syndicated on NBC/Talknet, broadcast on three hundred radio stations nationwide. Her next talk shows aired mid-morning on media giant WGY in Albany, New York, and then on WPRO, Providence, Rhode Island. Currently, in addition to seeing clients and writing a series of sex and astrology books, her astrology talk show is on WPRO, and she writes a weekly astrology column.

Her background is eclectic. Starting with a liberal arts education, she went on to earn a Bachelor of Fine Arts degree in painting from Rhode Island School of Design, spending her senior year in Italy on the European Honors' Program, and she speaks Italian fluently. While in college, she completed a year of equity apprenticeship at Trinity Repertory Theater in Rhode Island. She holds Master of Arts degrees in teaching and psychology and has taught art on every level from preschool through college—in private classes, public middle school, and at Rhode Island School of Design.

Myrna has been married to Robert Lamb for thirty-eight years. They have two beloved daughters and three grandchildren. They live in Lincoln, Rhode Island, in an early American home that they have faithfully restored.

Hampton Roads Publishing Company
. . . for the evolving human spirit

HAMPTON ROADS PUBLISHING COMPANY publishes books
on a variety of subjects, including metaphysics, spirituality,
health, visionary fiction, and other related topics.

For a copy of our latest trade catalog or consumer catalog,
call toll-free, 800-766-8009, or send your name and address to:

HAMPTON ROADS PUBLISHING COMPANY, INC.
1125 STONEY RIDGE ROAD · CHARLOTTESVILLE, VA 22902
e-mail: hrpc@hrpub.com · www.hrpub.com